# Equine
# Endoscopy and Arthroscopy

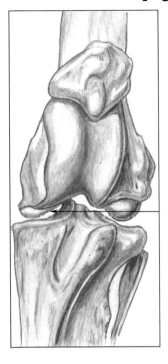

## for the
## Equine Practitioner

Sameeh M. Abutarbush, BVSc,
MVetSc, Diplomate ABVP,
Diplomate ACVIM

James L. Carmalt, MA, VetMB,
MVetSc, MRCVS, Diplomate
ABVP, Diplomate ACVS

Contributor:
Claire Card, DVM, PhD, Diplomate ACT

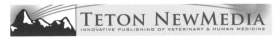
TETON NEWMEDIA
INNOVATIVE PUBLISHING OF VETERINARY & HUMAN MEDICINE

Jackson, Wyoming 83001

Executive Editor: Carroll C. Cann
Illustrations of the Arthroscopy and Respiratory Tract chapters: Kathryn Carmalt
AS, BSc, MSc
Illustrations of the Gastrointestinal and Urinary Tract chapters: Cori Forbes

Teton NewMedia
P.O. Box 4833
Jackson, WY 83001
1-888-770-3165
www.tetonnm.com

PRINTED IN THE UNITED STATES OF AMERICA

ISBN # 1-59161-039-7

Print number 5 4 3 2 1

Library of Congress Cataloging-in-Publication Data on file.

# Dedication

I would like to dedicate this book to my beloved parents, Mohammad Abutarbush and Fatima Abu-Kuhail, and my brothers and sisters, Nidal, Reem, Khaled, Mai, Omar and Mahmoud Abutarbush, who have helped me throughout my life, both personally and professionally. I could not have asked for a better, more patient, loving and caring family. Thank you!

Sameeh M. Abutarbush

I would like to dedicate this book to my parents, Lawrence and Inez, my brother David and to my loving wife Kathryn and daughter Jessica. They are outstanding people who have worked hard, made sacrifices, guided and lent me their unending support to allow me the opportunity to pursue the career of my dreams.

Dr. Ian and Mrs. Janet Keymer and Dr. "Tim" Cheyne introduced me to veterinary medicine, guided me through school and nurtured my ambitions. I hope that this book meets your expectations.

James L. Carmalt

# In Memory
# of a Great Mentor

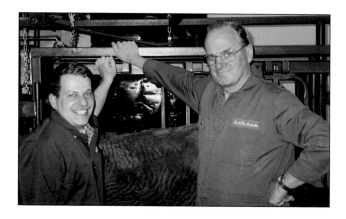

On December 15th, 2006 the veterinary profession lost a fine member and senior leader: Professor Otto M. Radostits. Professor Radostits was like a father to me during my internship and residency at The Western College of Veterinary Medicine, University of Saskatchewan, and had remained so until his death. Professor Radostits was a devoted mentor, an honest advisor, a phenomenal teacher and an excellent clinician. His love and enthusiasm for veterinary medicine is unprecedented.

Professor Radostits had a great influence on my life and career. He taught me how to write scientifically, be a dedicated teacher, and an observant clinician. I always remember him reminding me, while we were examining animals together, with his incredible booming voice and great smile, "Sameeh, you will make more mistakes not looking than not knowing".

Professor Otto M. Radostits died while he was battling cancer after he dedicated over forty years of his life to veterinary medicine.

I miss you so much and this book is in your memory; Professor Radostits.

Sameeh M. Abutarbush

# Acknowledgement

We would like to thank our colleagues at the Western College of Veterinary Medicine, University of Saskatchewan as well as the staff and veterinarians at Scone Veterinary Hospital for their help in collecting some of the endoscopic views used in this book.

Our residency supervisors played an enormous role in our professional development, for which we are eternally grateful.

In addition we would like to thank Carroll Cann from Teton NewMedia for his guidance in the development of this book and for his amazing personality!

Sameeh M. Abutarbush

James L. Carmalt

# Table of Contents

# Section 4 Endoscopy of the Guttural Pouch

# Section 5 Endoscopy of the Nasopharynx

# Section 6 Endoscopy of the Larynx

# Section 7 Endoscopy of the Trachea and Bronchi

# Section 8 Endoscopy of the Esophagus

# Section 9 Endoscopy of the Stomach

# Section 10 Endoscopy of the Duodenum

# Section 11 Endoscopy of the Urethra, Bladder and Ureters

# Section 12   Endoscopy of the Reproductive System of the Stallion

# Section 13   Endoscopy of the Reproductive System of the Mare

# Section 14 Arthroscopy

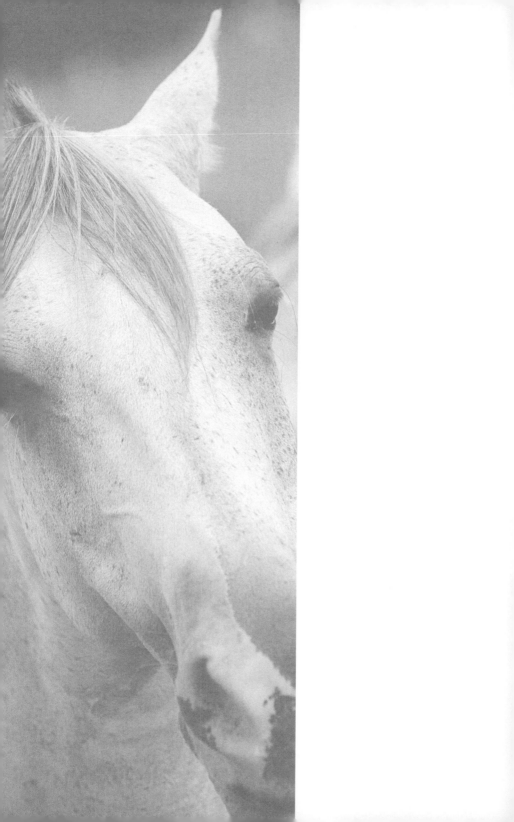

# Section 1

# Endoscopy Equipment, Use and Maintenance

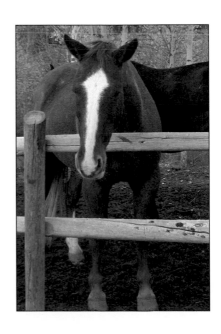

# General Principles

**The goal of this book** is to provide a manual of endoscopic technique and application for the equine practitioner. The emphasis is on commonly performed endoscopic procedures by body region including the joints. Normal anatomy, anatomic anomalies and abnormal clinical findings are clearly explained. Medical and surgical indications are provided and common procedural errors are highlighted throughout the text.

# Some Helpful Hints

Scattered throughout the text, you will find the following symbols to help you focus on what is routine and what may be really important:

✓ This is a routine feature or basic point for understanding the subject discussed.

♥ This is an important feature. You should remember this.

☞ The key symbol will be used selectively to indicate a very important point to assist your understanding of the topic area.

💣 Something serious will happen if you do not remember this, possibly resulting in injury or loss of the patient, and upset to the client.

3

There is a large range of endoscopic equipment available to the veterinary practitioner. This can range from the dedicated in-house system (Figure 1-1) to the general-purpose in-field system (Figure 1-2). These can be purchased new or in a reconditioned state from a variety of veterinary suppliers and online auction houses.

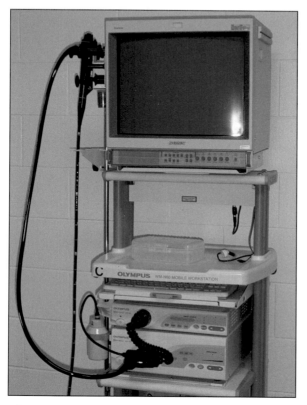

**Figure 1-1** Videoendoscope unit for in-house use. Monitor, light source and video unit, water supply.

✔ The main difference in these systems is that the in-house set-up consists of a videoendoscope attached to an integral light/power source whereas the in-field systems are usually fibreoptic and the image is viewed via an eyepiece rather than a television monitor. The integral system has the added benefit that images can be stored on videotape (digital or analogue) for further in-depth study after the endoscopic procedure has been completed. Most of the pictures in this book were obtained using the endoscopy unit depicted in Figure 1-1. Images were then stored either on a VHS or digital video system.

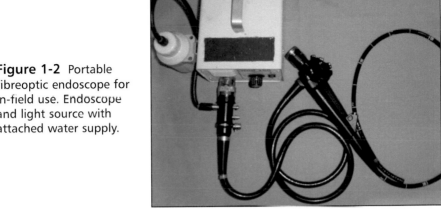

**Figure 1-2** Portable fibreoptic endoscope for in-field use. Endoscope and light source with attached water supply.

✓ There are two common methods of holding the body of the endoscope, the "under-hand" (Figure 1-3) and the "over-hand" technique (Figure 1-4). The authors strongly recommend the latter method as it allows for fine adjustment with minimal extraneous movement and is ultimately more comfortable for the operator. Additionally, the use of the over-hand technique results in a better grasp of the equipment in the event of an accident.

It is preferable to have a working knowledge of the endoscope, prior to clinical use (Figure 1-5).

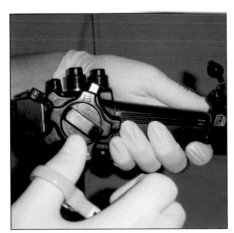

**Figure 1-3** The under-hand technique.

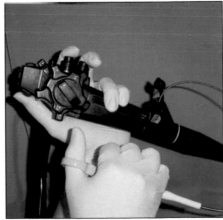

**Figure 1-4** The over-hand-technique. Note the ability of the user to utilize all hand-controls and the biopsy instrument with a single hand, while maintaining a good grasp of the control body.

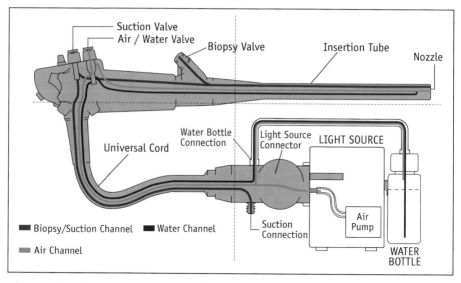

**Figure 1-5** A cut-away diagram of a common Olympus endoscope
Picture courtesy of Olympus Australia.

♥ This is especially important when the biopsy channel is to be used, for example for a guide wire (during entry into the guttural pouches). As can be seen in Figure 1-6, the biopsy channel is eccentrically placed and thus when viewing an image on the video screen the instrument is seen to appear to the immediate left of the endoscopic view (9 o'clock). While the importance of this is not immediately apparent, this will affect the technique employed during certain procedures (please see guttural pouch endoscopy, Page 33).

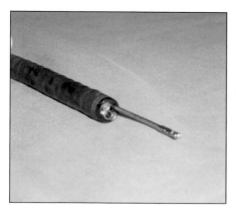

**Figure 1-6** The distal end of an endo-scope. Note the eccentric placement of the biopsy channel.

♥ Assuming that the endoscope has been placed in the correct position, one of the most common mistakes made by endoscope users is to fail to place the area of interest in the center of the field-of-view, or to inadvertently rotate the endoscope, thus rotating the image. This has the unwanted side effect of having the audience unconsciously tip their heads in order to make sense of the image. This is amusing to bystanders but does little to improve the diagnostic usefulness of the subsequent image!

♥ Endoscope maintenance is often neglected and yet is extremely important to the longevity of the equipment as well as to reduce the likelihood of transmitting communicable diseases between horses. Endoscopes should be cleaned using an enzymatic detergent (flushed and brushed) following each procedure. This is to prevent drying of fibrin or purulent material and clogging of the working channels. Disinfection should follow using complete immersion in chemicals, such as sodium perborate (PeraSafe®), compatible with the endoscope. The instrument should be subsequently rinsed and the channels flushed with alcohol to facilitate drying. Manufacturers' guidelines on endoscope cleaning should be followed. Automated endoscope washers/disinfectors are also available.

✓ Additional equipment for endoscopic procedures can include guide wires, biopsy, rat-toothed and basket forceps as well as snares (Figure 1-7).

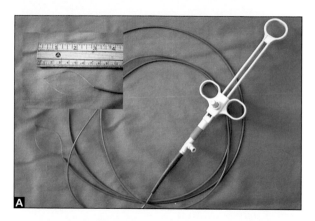

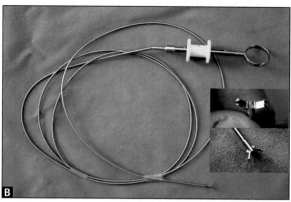

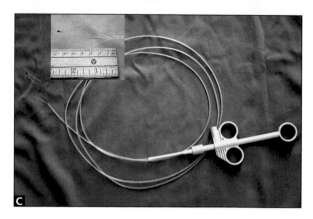

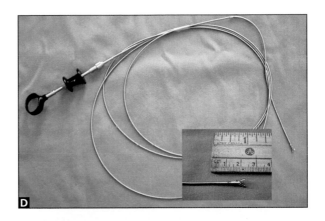

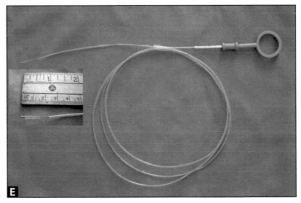

**Figure 1-7A-E** A = Snare; B= Toothed Forceps; C= Basket Forceps; D= Biopsy Forceps; E= Brush.

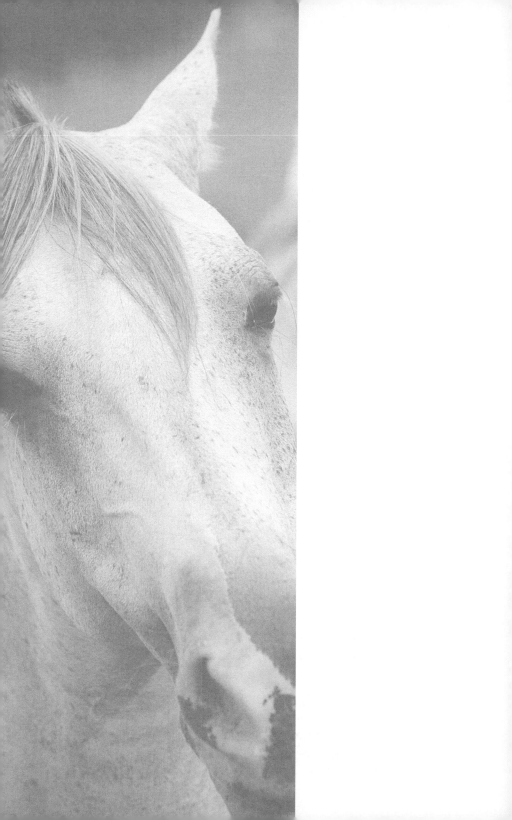

# Section 2

# Endoscopy of the Nasal Passages

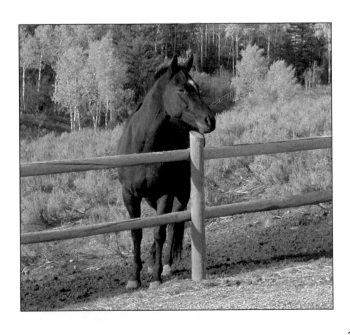

# Anatomy

The nasal passages encompass the region from immediately rostral to the nasopharynx to the external nares, including the nasomaxillary opening but not the sinuses.

The nasal septum divides the nares into left and right nostrils.

Each nostril is comprised of a dorsal, middle and ventral meatus. These divisions are a function of the rostral extension of the dorsal conchal and ventral conchal sinuses (Figure 2-1) with the ventral meatus being the widest, followed by the middle and lastly the dorsal which is relatively narrow.

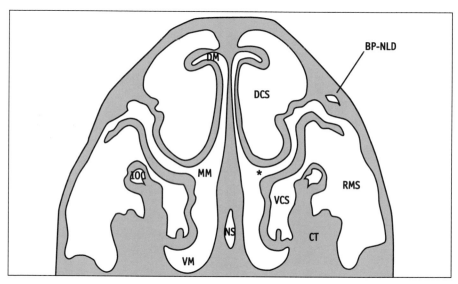

**Figure 2-1** A cross-section of the maxilla (mid-facial crest) showing the anatomy of the rostral extensions of the sinus and division of the nasal cavity. DCS – Dorsal Conchal Sinus, VCS – Ventral Conchal Sinus, RMS – Rostral maxillary sinus, CT – Cheek tooth, BP-NLP – Bony portion of the Nasolacrymal duct, IOC – Infraorbital canal, VM – Ventral meatus, MM – Middle meatus, DM – Dorsal meatus, NS – Nasal septum * – Nasomaxillary opening.

# Clinical Signs of Nasal Passage Disease

✓ Clinical signs can include:

• Unilateral nasal discharge.

- Stertorous breathing.
- Unilateral facial deformation.
- Fetid odor.

# Endoscopic Technique

Dependent on the area of interest:

✓ Dorsal meatus only for the ethmoidal bones (Figure 2-2).

✓ Middle meatus for nasomaxillary opening (Figure 2-3).

✓ Ventral meatus for nasopharynx, guttural pouches and tracheal examination.

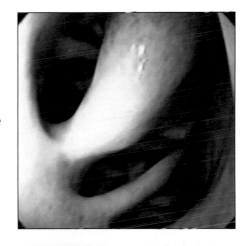

**Figure 2-2** Endoscopic view of the normal dorsal meatus extension of the ethmoid labyrinth.

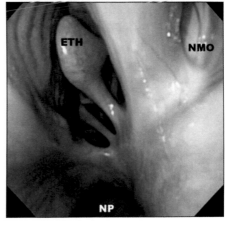

**Figure 2-3** Endoscope placement within the left middle meatus. Note the ethmoids dorsally (ETH) the normal nasomaxillary opening to the right (NMO) and the nasopharynx (NP).

13

♥ Ensuring the endoscope is placed in the ventral meatus is achieved by placing the index finger on the endoscope tip and directing it medially and ventrally into the meatus.

🖐 It is important to remember that the nasal passages are the most rostral extension of the respiratory tract and thus the presence of foreign material (feed, purulent debris) must be interpreted in light of other endoscopic findings, before automatically assigning the abnormality specifically to the nares (Figures 2-4 and 2-5).

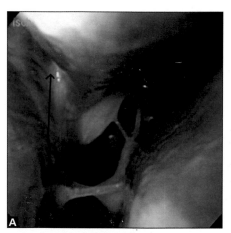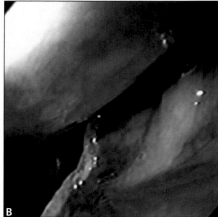

**Figure 2-4A,B** The presence of purulent material in the region of the nasomaxillary opening (arrow) in the middle meatus of this horse is due to coughing. The horse had a lower airway disease and no evidence of sinusitis (A). The purulent material at the nasomaxillary opening in Figure 4B is of a horse with sinusitis.

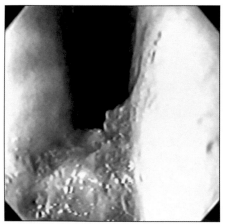

**Figure 2-5** The presence of feed material in the nares can be an indicator of dysphagia due to an undetermined cause.

# Diseases of the Nasal Passages

## Rhinitis

**Allergic:**

Uncommon.

Hypersensitivity reaction to inhaled allergens.

✓ Often the inciting cause cannot be determined.

✓ Clinical signs include acute onset nasal discharge and congestion with labored breathing and dyspnea (Figure 2-6).

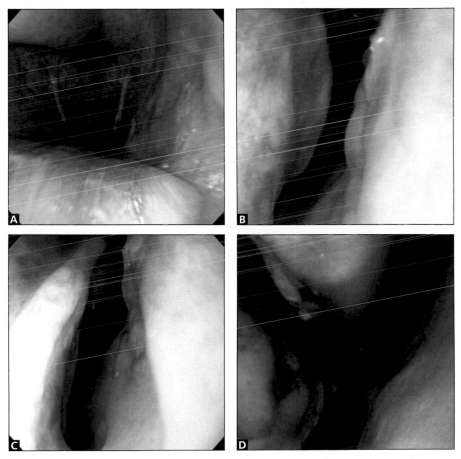

**Figure 2-6A-D** Endoscopic views of the nasopharynx (A), caudal ventral meatus (B), rostral ventral meatus (C) and middle meatus (D) of a horse with allergic rhinitis. Note the discharge, edema and hyperemia of the mucosa.

**Fungal:**

✓ *Aspergillus spp.* but others including *Mucor spp.* or *Candida spp.* may be involved.

✓ *Coccidiomycosis immitis*, *Histoplasma* and *Cryptococcus* infection have also been reported.

✓ Significant soft tissue destruction ensues in areas of damaged or necrotic tissue, in other cases, spontaneous infection appears to occur (Figure 2-7).

✓ Clinical signs vary and can range from nothing to halitosis, nasal discharge and headshaking.

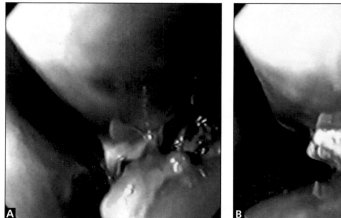
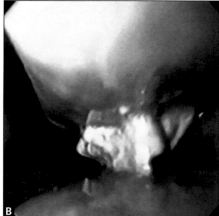

**Figure 2-7A,B** Endoscopic view of the middle meatus of a horse affected with fungal rhinitis. Note the presence of the fungal plaque and associated mucus.

# Nasal Septum Deviation / Inflammation

Traumatic thickening, abscess formation, hamartoma (abnormal formation of normal tissue), neoplasia and cystic degeneration have all been reported in the horse.

✓ Irrespective of the cause, most lesions will require surgical resection to resolve the clinical signs of facial distortion, stertor or complete obstruction of the nasal passages.

✓ These lesions can be quite difficult to appreciate on endoscopy, unless narrowing of the nasal passages has occurred to the extent that passage of the instrument is impeded.

✓ Radiography is a useful adjunct modality in these cases.

# Ethmoid Hematoma

Unknown cause.

✓ Hemorrhage between laminae of submucosa leads to fibrosis, further bleeding and mass expansion.

✓ Clinical signs include intermittent, mild, unilateral epistaxis and usually there is no obstruction to airflow until expansion into the nasal cavity occurs.

✓ In early cases there may be no visible lesion endoscopically.

Vary in color from a red/yellow to a deep red/green color. (Figure 2-8).

Treatment:

- Intralesional formalin injection.
- Cryotherapy.
- Laser excision.

Surgical debulking:

- Recurrence rate is approximately 40%, irrespective of treatment modality.

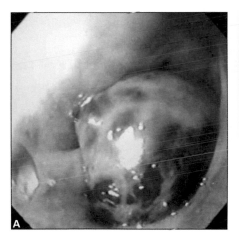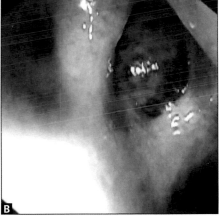

**Figure 2-8A,B** Ethmoid hematomas can vary in color (A, B). Only the rostral extent can be seen at the limit of the ethmoidal labyrinth but extends caudally and may also involve one or both maxillary sinuses (see page 28).

# Fungal Infection of the Ethmoid Labyrinth

✓ Initiated by trauma or spontaneous infection (Figure 2-9).

✓ Etiological agent = A. *fumigatus*.

✓ Incidence unknown.

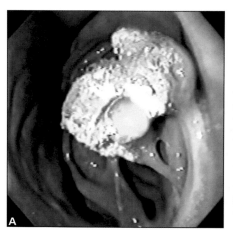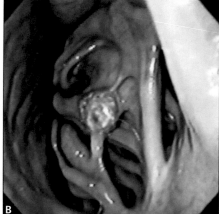

**Figure 2-9A,B** Fungal infection of the ethmoid labyrinth pre (A) and post (B) treatment. An incidental finding following repeated nasogastric intubation.

# Neoplastic Masses

✓ Most neoplastic masses within the nares are the result of extension of a mass from a remote region e.g.: ethmoidal hematoma or sinus disease (Figure 2-10).

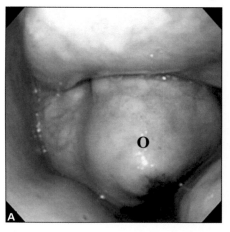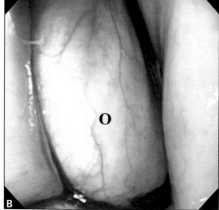

**Figure 2-10A,B** Expansion of an osteoma from the nasal bones extending ventrally into the nasal passages. (O = Osteoma)

✓ Eosinophilic granulomas, squamous cell carcinoma have been diagnosed as originating within the nasal cavity.

# Miscellaneous Diseases

✓ While feed within the nasal passages is usually due to dysphagia (Figure 2-5), in some cases (Figures 2-11 and 2-12) it is due to an oroantral fistula.

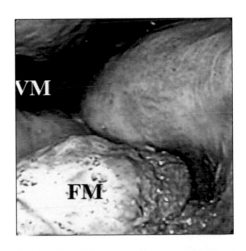

**Figure 2-11** A mass of feed material within the left ventral meatus of the nose. Courtesy of Dr. Michael Lowder. (VM = Ventral Meatus, FM = Feed Mass)

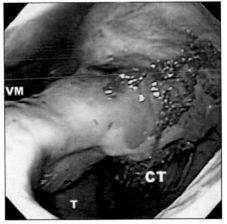

**Figure 2-12** Having removed the feed material an oroantral fistula can be seen. Note the ventral meatus (VM), tongue (T) and cheek tooth (CT). Courtesy of Dr. Michael Lowder.

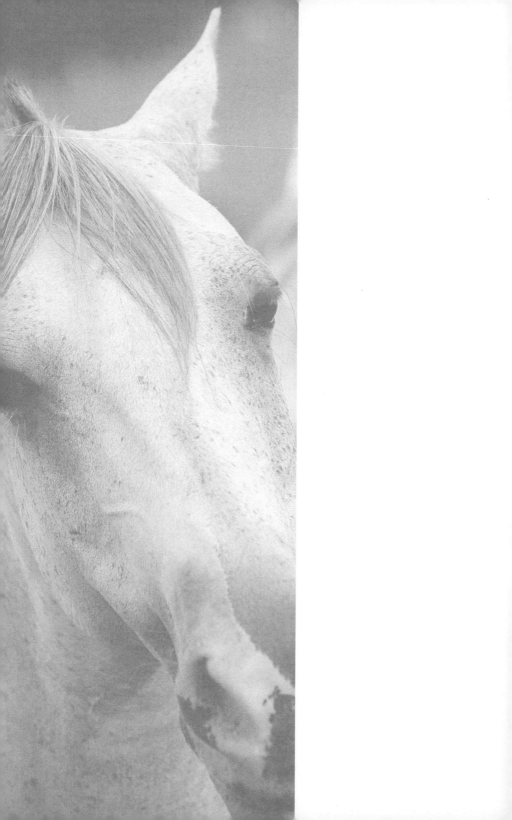

# Section 3

# Endoscopy of the Paranasal Sinuses

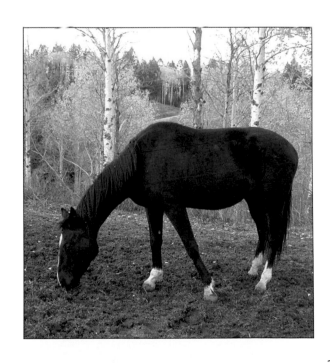

# Anatomy

Six pairs of paranasal sinuses (Figures 2-1, 3-1 through 3-3):

- Rostral maxillary
- Ventral conchal
- Dorsal conchal
- Frontal
- Caudal maxillary
- Sphenopalatine

✓ Some authors include the ethmoid sinus as part of the paranasal sinus system. However this system is blood-filled, not air-filled, as with the remainder of the commonly cited sinuses.

Caudal portions of the dorsal conchal sinus and the rostral portion of the frontal sinus are collectively referred to as the dorsoconchal sinus in some texts.

✓ The dorsal conchal and frontal sinuses communicate with the caudal maxillary sinus via the frontomaxillary opening. Ultimately sinuses drain into the middle meatus of the nasal passages via the nasomaxillary opening.

✓ In rare cases the sphenopalatine sinus may have a direct communication with the nasopharynx.

Rostral maxillary and ventral conchal sinuses communicate over the infraorbital canal.

Rostral maxillary / ventral conchal sinuses are maintained distinct from the caudal maxillary sinus system by a complete bony septum which may be destroyed by disease

✓ The caudal roots of cheek tooth 3 and cheek tooth 4 reside in the rostral maxillary sinus. Cheek teeth 5 and 6 are contained within the caudal maxillary sinus.

✓ Due to mesial drift, the exact position of the teeth needs to be determined with accuracy during disease investigation.

**Figure 3-1** Dorsolateral view of the paranasal sinus system in an anatomical specimen.
FS – Frontal Sinus, DCS – Dorsal Conchal Sinus, ETH – Ethmoid Sinus, VCS – Ventral Conchal Sinus, RMS – Rostral Maxillary Sinus, CMS – Caudal Maxillary Sinus, IOC – Infraorbital canal, * – Bony Septum between RMS & CMS.

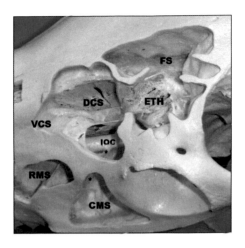

**Figure 3-2** Dorsoventral view of the paranasal sinus system in an anatomical specimen.
FS – Frontal Sinus, DCS – Dorsal Conchal Sinus, ETH – Ethmoid Sinus, RMS – Rostral Maxillary Sinus, BP–NLD - Bony portion of the Nasolacrymal duct.
Cross-hatch = Removed caudal extension of rostral maxillary sinus.
Stippling = Area of frontomaxillary opening.

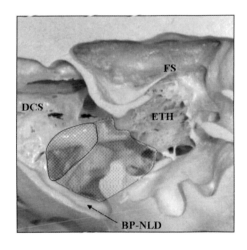

**Figure 3-3** Lateral view of the paranasal sinus system in an anatomical specimen.
FS – Frontal Sinus, DCS – Dorsal Conchal Sinus, ETH – Ethmoid Sinus, RMS – Rostral Maxillary Sinus, CMS – Caudal Maxillary Sinus, IOC – Infraorbital canal, * – Bony Septum between RMS & CMS.

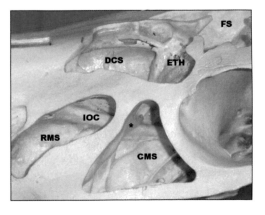

# Endoscopic Technique

✔ Endoscopic examination of the paranasal sinus system can be performed on a standing sedated horse or under general anesthesia.

✔ A rigid arthroscope or flexible endoscope can be used to examine the paranasal sinuses each with a distinct benefit.

♥ The rigid arthroscope requires a smaller access portal and has a wider field of view, which is important in an area with limited space, especially if diseased. However, other than rotating the arthroscope to utilize the 30 degree angulation (or greater if a 70 degree arthroscope is available), care must be taken during movement to avoid damage to portal margins. Another disadvantage is that the lens cannot be cleaned while within the sinus.

♥ The flexible endoscope requires a larger portal than the arthroscope. It is useful because cleaning of the lens is possible (using attached fluids) and there is greater mobility with little, if any, collateral damage to portal margins.

✔ Portals can be created using an appropriately sized Steinmann pin, drill bit or Michelle trephine.

The horse is sedated according to standard practices and a small amount of local anesthetic agent is placed subcutaneously to the level of the periosteum in the required site. A stab incision is made through the skin and periosteum to the underlying bone. The skin edges are separated using a small hemostat and the perforating instrument is placed perpendicular to the bone surface. Controlled access to the sinuses is made.

✔ Be aware that the horse may move as the sinus is perforated because the underlying mucosa has not been subjected to local anesthesia. This is not usually a problem however the horse handler and veterinarian should be aware of the possible danger.

Portal placement for access to the various sinus systems are as follows (Figure 3-4):

Frontal Sinus

Midway between the supraorbital foramen and the midline.

Caudal Maxillary Sinus

2 cm rostral and 1cm ventral to the medial canthus of the eye.

Rostral Maxillary Sinus

Half way along, and 4 cm ventral to a line connecting the medial canthus of the eye to the nasoincisive notch (the path of the bony portion of the Nasolacrymal duct).

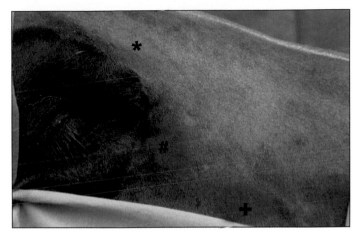

**Figure 3-4** Portal Positioning for Sinus Endoscopy.
\* = Frontal Sinus; # = Caudal Maxillary Sinus; + = Rostral Maxillary Sinus.

# Endoscopic Anatomy

Endoscopic anatomy of a normal equine (cadaver) sinus can be found in Figures 3-5 through 3-8. Please refer to gross anatomy (Figures 3-1 to 3-3) for a greater understanding of this challenging region.

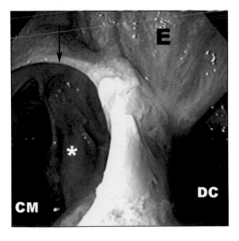

**Figure 3-5** Endoscopic view of the frontal sinus (caudal view) showing the dorsal conchal, (DC), ethmoid (E) and caudal maxillary (CM) sinuses, the frontomaxillary opening (arrow) and the third molar tooth (\*).

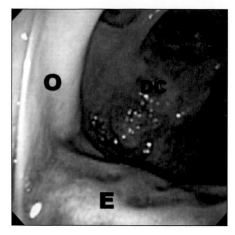

**Figure 3-6** Endoscopic view of the frontal sinus (cranial view) showing the dorsal conchal sinus (ahead, DC), ethmoid (below, E) and abaxial wall of the orbit (left, O).

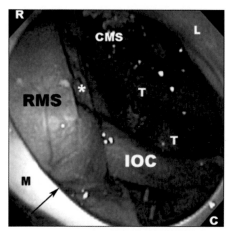

**Figure 3-7** Endoscopic view from within the frontal sinus (ventral view) showing the fronto-maxillary opening (arrow), tooth roots (T) within the caudal maxillary sinus (CMS), the thin bulla of the caudodorsal portion of the rostral maxillary sinus (RMS) and the infraorbital canal (IOC). R = Rostral, C = Caudal, L= Lateral, M= Medial. Note the iatrogenic damage to the bulla in this cadaver specimen (*).

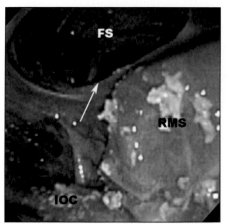

**Figure 3-8** Endoscopic view of the rostral portion of the caudal maxillary sinus. Frontomaxillary opening (top, arrow), the frontal sinus, infraorbital canal (IOC) and thin bulla of the caudodorsal portion of the rostral maxillary sinus (RMS) with bone spicules from a previous frontal sinoscopy portal in this cadaver specimen.

Limitations:

✔ By the time that the horse is presented for veterinary examination the sinuses are often filled with fluid, purulent material or soft tissue.

✔ In the former cases, a sinus flush to expel the offending material is often of benefit to enable visualization of the disease process.

✔ Soft tissue masses often require biopsy for definitive diagnosis.

✔ Biopsy samples can be obtained endoscopically, however obtaining diagnostic samples often requires a sinusotomy thus negating minimally invasive endoscopic evaluation of the sinus.

✔ Portal Placement.

✔ In cases where the surgeon wishes to retain a bone flap for closure of a sinusotomy, the placement of a trephine hole for endoscope placement may weaken the flap to the extent that it fractures during the sinusotomy procedure. As long as the periosteum is retained however, this is not likely to result in a problem.

# Diseases of the Sinuses

## Primary and Secondary Sinusitis

Primary sinusitis·

✔ Associated with upper respiratory infection, especially in young horses.

✔ Transitory and self-limiting in most cases unless inflammation leads to swelling of the mucosal lining and closure of the nasomaxillary opening.

✔ Fungal sinusitis in older horses may present with intermittent epistaxis of undetermined origin. Endoscopy of the nasal passages may indicate the presence of blood or fungal plaque at the nasomaxillary opening, in some cases. In other cases there are no endoscopic abnormalities. Sinoscopy in these cases can be rewarding (Figure 3-9).

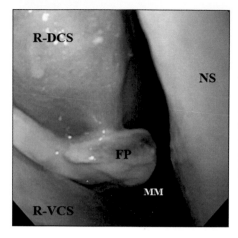

**Figure 3-9** A fungal plaque invading the middle meatus from the nasomaxillary opening in a case of fungal sinusitis. (R – DCS = Rostral Extension of Dorsal Conchal Sinus) (R – VCS = Rostral Extension of Ventral Conchal Sinus) NS = Nasal Septum FP = Fungal Plaque, MM = Middle Meatus)

Secondary sinusitis:

The most common cause of clinically apparent sinus disease.

✓ Associated with periapical infection of the cheek teeth.

Diagnosis:

• Fetid nasal discharge with or without facial swelling depending on the patency of the nasomaxillary opening.

✓ Response (decreased drainage) to antimicrobial therapy which recurs following cessation of treatment.

✓ Radiographs have a low specificity and sensitivity for dental disease. A combination of nuclear scintigraphy and radiography improves diagnostic ability.

✓ Sinoscopic visualization of the tooth apex may allow definitive diagnosis.

# Neoplasia

Squamous cell carcinoma.

Amelioblastoma and Odontoma.

# Ethmoid Hematoma

✓ Sinoscopic examination is indicated to confirm the extension of ethmoid hematomas beyond the limit of nasal visualization.

✓ Intralesional formalin treatment can be performed sinoscopically. See page 17.

# Paranasal Sinus Cyst

A common abnormality specifically in young horses.

Diagnosis:

✓ Facial swelling, often in the absence of fetid nasal discharge.

✓ Radiographically, there is an absence of gas within the sinus which may be filled with a soft tissue/fluid radiodensity.

✓ Clear fluid egress immediately following trephination.

✓ Sinoscopically, the fluid is clear and yellow with crystalline particulate material which can be seen to glisten in the light of the instrument.

✓ Visualization of normal anatomical landmarks within the sinus system can be difficult.

# Fractures and Trauma

✓ Visualization of the bony portion of the nasolacrymal duct may be of use in cases where facial fractures are thought to have disrupted the integrity of the duct.

✓ Direct assessment of facial fractures in the region of the paranasal sinuses is not possible, without mucosal compromise, as the entire sinus has a respiratory mucosal lining (Figures 3-10, 3-11, 3-12 and 3-13).

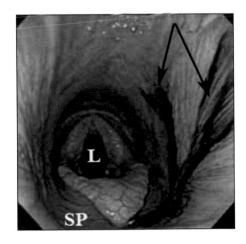

**Figure 3-10** Endoscopic view of the nasopharynx in a case of epistaxis of undetermined origin. Note pooling of blood (arrows) on the soft palate (SP). L – Larynx.

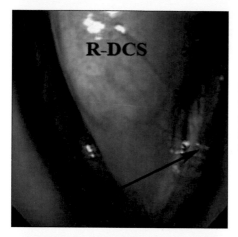

**Figure 3-11** Endoscopic view of the nasomaxillary opening in the middle meatus. Note the presence of blood (arrow) in this region. R-DCS – Rostral extension of the dorsal conchal sinus.

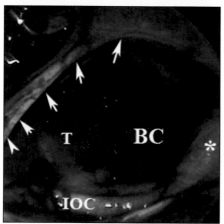

**Figure 3-12** Sinoscopic view of the same horse (above). Rostral and lateral are to the right and top respectively. BC- Blood clot, IOC – Infraorbital canal, T-Tooth root, * – Caudal extension of the rostral maxillary sinus. The limits of the frontomaxillary opening are delineated by arrows.

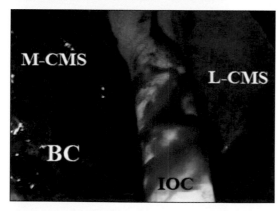

**Figure 3-13** Sinoscopic view of the same horse looking caudally. Lateral (L – CMS) and medial (M – CMS) caudal maxillary sinus, divided by the infraorbital canal (IOC). Note the presence of the blood clot (BC). This was a case of acute trauma. No fractures were seen.

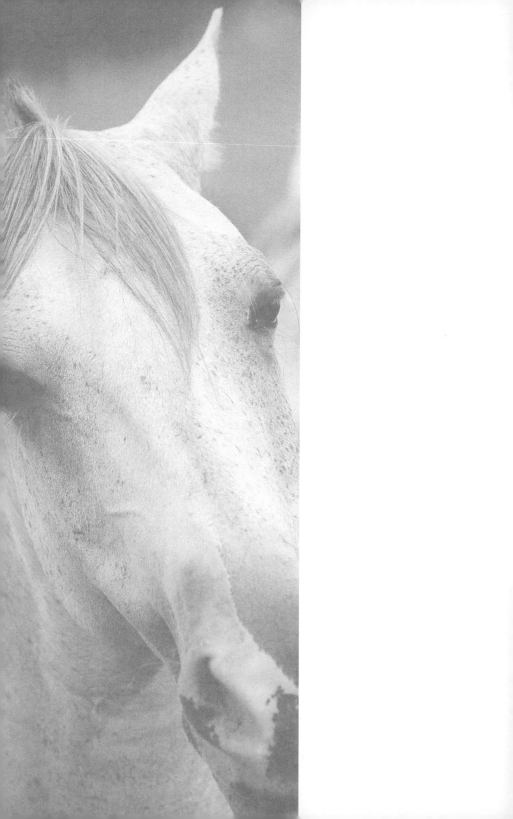

# Section 4

# Endoscopy of the Guttural Pouch

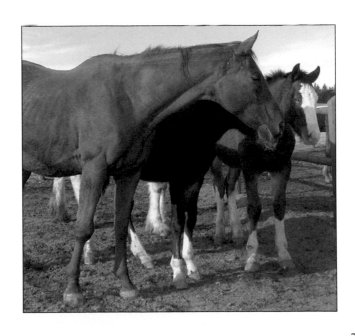

*Endoscopy of both guttural pouches is an integral component of a complete upper airway examination.*

# Anatomy

Guttural pouches are air-filled diverticuli of the auditory tubes.

They are located in the caudal area of the head; extend from the roof of the pharynx to the base of the skull and from the atlanto-occipital joint to the pharyngeal recess.

Pouches communicate with the nasopharynx and open routinely during swallowing (Figure 4-1).

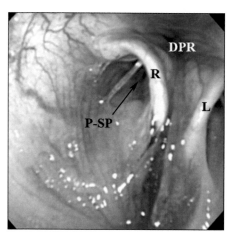

**Figure 4-1** Endoscopic view of the nasopharynx during swallowing showing the concurrent guttural pouch opening. (DPR – Dorsal pharyngeal recess, L-Left, R-Right, P-SP – Plica-Salpingopharyngea)

✓ Volume of each pouch is approximately 600ml; divided into two compartments (medial and lateral) by the stylohyoid bone.

✓ The stylohyoid bone articulates dorsally with the petrous temporal bone and is covered by a thin strip of muscle rostrally. This is the stylopharyngeus muscle.

## The Medial Compartment

✓ 2/3 of the total volume.

⚷ The glossopharyngeal (CRN IX), vagus (CRN X) and the hypoglossal (CRN XII) nerves travel in a fold of mucosa lying caudo-medial to the internal carotid artery.

⚷ The sympathetic trunk, cranio-cervical ganglion, cranial laryngeal nerve (branch of CRN X) and the accessory-spinal nerve (CRN XI) travel in another mucosal fold, which in most horses is intimately associated with the artery.

✓ The pharyngeal branches of CRN IX and X travel in a rostro-ventral direction along the lateral and medial walls of the medial compartment until interdigitating in a plexus of nerve fibers covering the surface of the floor of the medial compartment.

☞ Under the floor of the medial compartment, the swelling of the retropharyngeal lymph node can be appreciated. The nerve plexus serves to innervate the soft palate and thus any pathological process in this compartment has the potential to affect pharyngeal function.

## The Lateral Compartment

✓ 1/3 of the total volume.

✓ External carotid artery passes from craniomedial to caudolateral bifurcating into the superficial temporal and the maxillary arteries.

✓ The maxillary-facial vein is present and the facial nerve (CRN VII) exits the skull via the stylomastoid foramen traveling across the dorsal surface of the lateral pouch.

# Endoscopic Technique

Place endoscope in ventral meatus of nose (Figure 4-2).

✓ Placement in middle meatus makes pouch entry difficult as pharyngeal openings slope caudoventrally and the tip of the endoscope may slip into the caudal nasopharynx when entry is attempted (Figure 4-3).

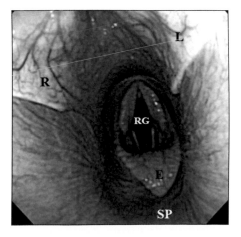

**Figure 4-2** Normal nasopharynx from the ventral meatus: GP openings (L-Left and R-right), soft palate (SP), epiglottis (E) and rima glottis (RG).

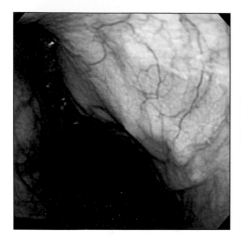

**Figure 4-3** Middle meatus placement: Note position relative to GP opening. (See also Figure 4-16)

✔ Examine meati, nasomaxillary opening of the paranasal sinuses, ethmoidal bones, nasopharynx, larynx and dorsopharyngeal recess prior to guttural pouch entry.

✔ An initial examination of the nasopharynx is performed prior to entering the pharyngeal orifice.

This allows the investigator to assess the shape of the lateral and dorsal pharyngeal wall as well as the openings themselves. Distention of the pouches (with air or fluid) can lead to compression of the nasopharynx as the lateral walls are moved medially by the distention.

Fluid, blood or mucoid material can be visualized exiting the affected pouch.

# Entry into the Pouches (using a biopsy stylette)

✔ **Left:** The biopsy channel position is to the left of the viewing lens and light source. Advancement of the endoscope into the guttural pouch is achieved by levering the cartilaginous flap open and since the endoscope biopsy channel position is to the left of the viewing lens and light source, simply advancing the biopsy instrument into the left pouch opens the flap enough for endoscope entry.

✔ **Right:** Due to the position of the biopsy portal relative to the guttural pouch opening, advancing the biopsy instrument into the right guttural pouch simply places it along the lateral wall of the nasopharynx and therefore positioning the wire into the pouch followed by anti-clockwise rotation of the endoscope is usually necessary prior to advancing into the pouch (Figure 4-4A, B and C).

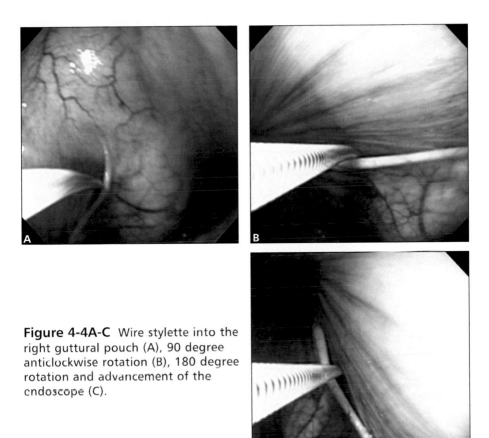

**Figure 4-4A-C** Wire stylette into the right guttural pouch (A), 90 degree anticlockwise rotation (B), 180 degree rotation and advancement of the endoscope (C).

# Entry into the Pouches (using an artificial insemination pipette)

♥ The end of a standard artificial insemination pipette is bent to approximately 30 degrees. This is placed up the nostril opposite the endoscope. Under endoscopic guidance, the pipette is advanced and rotated until the tip is underneath the guttural pouch opening on the endoscope side. Further rotation of the pipette will lift the medial lamina away from the wall of the nasopharynx and allow advancement of the endoscope into the pouch.

Once within the pharyngeal orifice, careful passage in a caudo-dorsal direction will allow visualization of the plica salpingopharyngea.

♥ This membranous structure marks the rostral extent of the eustation tube. The J-shaped structure leaves the lateral wall of the pharyngeal orifice and crosses the midline halfway up the pharyngeal opening forming a continuous ventral connection between the medial lamina of the eustation tube and the lateral wall of the pharynx (Figure 4-5). Passage of the endoscope beyond this point may result in air escaping from the pouch (in cases of tympany, Figure 4-10).

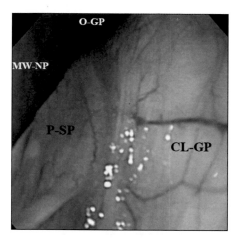

**Figure 4-5** Entrance to the right guttural pouch: Medial wall of nasopharynx (MW-NP) opening of the guttural pouch (O-GP), plica salpingopharyngea (P-SP) and cartilage lamina of the guttural pouch (CL-GP).

✔ Once within the pouch, retroflexion of the endoscope allows visualization of the caudal aspect of the plica, the insertion of the levator veli palatini muscle and the rostro-medial face of the guttural pouch. Other anatomical structures can be visualized as below (Figures 4-6 through 4-9- Left guttural pouch).

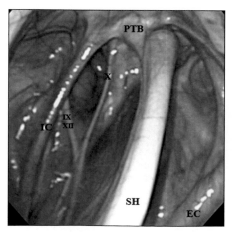

**Figure 4-6** Normal anatomy Medial compartment (left) divided from the lateral compartment (right) by the Stylohyoid bone (SH) articulating with the petrous portion of the temporal bone (PTB). Cranial nerves IX, X, XII, the internal carotid (IC) and external carotid (EC) arteries.

**Figure 4-7** Stylopharyngeus muscle (SP-M) overlies the stylohyoid bone (SH). The external carotid (EC) its extension, the external maxillary (EM) artery in the lateral compartment (Lateral). The internal carotid artery (IC) and the longus capitis and longus capitis ventralis (LC) muscles within the medial compartment (Medial).

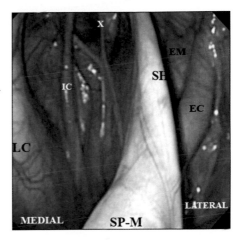

**Figure 4-8** Medial compartment: Straight muscles of the neck (longus capitis (LC) and longus capitis ventralis (LCV) internal carotid artery (IC), stylohyoid bone (SH), pharyngeal branches of cranial nerves IX (P-IX) and X (P-X).

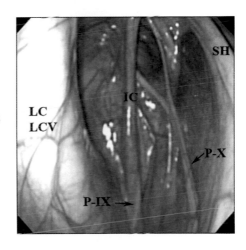

**Figure 4-9** Ramification of the pharyngeal branches of CRN IX (P-IX) and CRN X (P-X) occurs under the floor of the medial compartment (F-MC). The retropharyngeal lymph node lies directly under this nerve plexus. SP-M-Stylopharyngeus muscle.

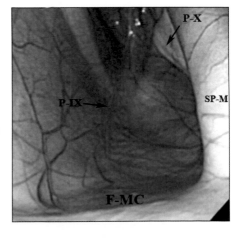

# Diseases of the Guttural Pouch

## Tympany

✓ Usually a disease of young foals.

Etiology unknown–A manifestation of a true plical disease (acting as a one-way valve) or a neural problem associated with inflammation.

✓ Presenting signs include:

- Dyspnea.
- Dysphagia.
- Uni-or bilateral swellings in the throat-latch region (Figure 4-10).

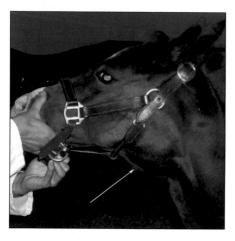

**Figure 4-10** A weanling foal with unilateral throat-latch swelling due to guttural pouch tympany (arrow).

✓ Endoscopic Signs can Include:

- Bulging of the walls of the Nasopharynx (Figure 4-11).
- Dorsal Pharyngeal collapse (Figure 4-12).
- Abnormal open position of guteral pouch openings (Figure 4-13).
- Dorsal displacement of the soft palate (Figure 4-16).

Intrapouch findings may include an increased amount of mucus, or no discernable abnormality.

✓ Treatment involves medial septum fenestration – Post treatment can look like Figure 4-20B (in unilateral cases or resection of the plica salpingopharyngeosa / GP osteum (in bilateral cases).

**Figure 4-11** Nasopharyngeal view of the guttural pouch openings in a case of tympany. Note: Left guttural pouch is bulging towards the midline (arrow) and concurrent pharyngitis (*).

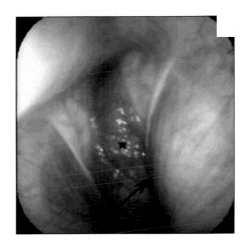

**Figure 4-12** Nasopharyngeal view in a case of guttural pouch tympany: Severe swelling of both pouches has resulted in dorsal collapse of the nasopharynx.

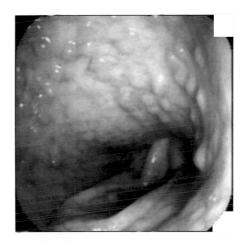

**Figure 4-13** Guttural pouch tympany: Note the abnormal open position of the cartilaginous opening due to extreme internal pressure.

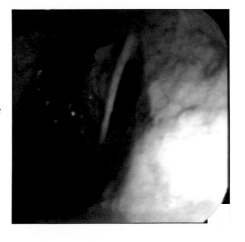

# Mycosis

✓ Clinical Signs:

  • Dependent on stage and location of the lesion.

  • Range from epistaxis (Figure 4-14), to dysphagia, dorsal displacement of the soft palate (Figure 4-16), to no appreciable clinical abnormality (Figure 4-20 below – medial septum plaque).

**Note:**

  ♥ In some cases, normal architecture of the guttural pouch may not be visible due to complete filling of the lumen by clotted blood (Figure 4-15, 4-17).

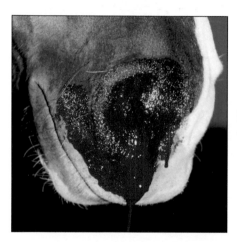

**Figure 4-14** Epistaxis in a clinical case of guttural pouch mycosis.

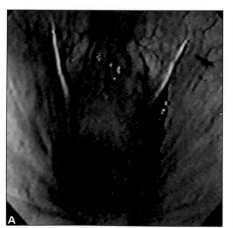
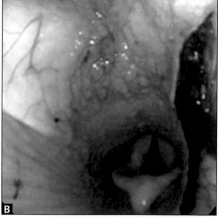

**Figure 4-15A,B** Blood clot protruding into the nasopharynx from the left guttural pouch (mycosis).

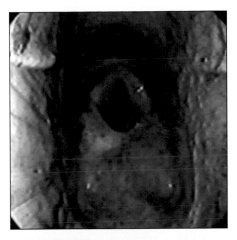

**Figure 4-16** Clinical signs of dysphagia associated with guttural pouch mycosis: Dorsal displacement of the soft palate and feed material immediately rostral to the caudal free border of the soft palate (Note: Inadvertent endoscope placement in the middle meatus).

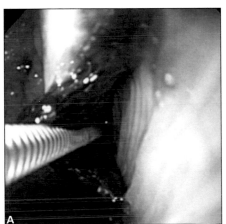 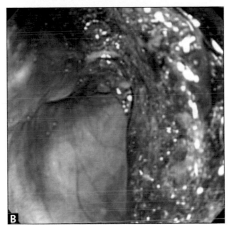

**Figure 4-17A,B** Left Guttural Pouch Mycosis with blood clot: Careful placement of biopsy stylette (left), Ventral portion of the medial compartment (Note: large blood clot dorsally, right).

⚷ It is *extremely* important not to disturb a blood clot within a guttural pouch. Exsanguination may follow.

♥ The ONLY reported differential diagnosis for this endoscopic finding is rupture of the ventral straight muscles of the neck – usually associated with trauma. Rupture of abscess-like lesion from these muscles may also cause significant epistaxis.

The fungal infection of the guttural pouch classically caudodorsal, overlying the internal carotid artery and inducing neuropraxia by virtue of the position (Figure 4-18).

Other reported positions of this plaque are on the stylohyoid bone (Figure 4-19), overlying the maxillary and superficial temporal arteries and on the medial septum between the pouches (Figure 4-20).

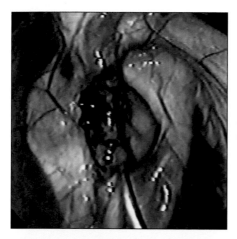

**Figure 4-18** Caudodorsal position of a mycotic plaque overlying the internal carotid artery.

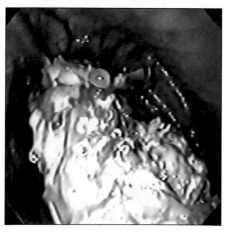

**Figure 4-19** Severe mycotic lesion covering the stylohyoid bone.

✓ *Aspergillus fumigatus* is the most common etiological agent.

✓ Fungal spores in a guttural pouch wash is not uncommon (due to the normal communication with the nasal passages), however the trigger mechanism facilitating colonization of the pouch remains uncertain.

✓ Some authors believe a blood substrate (vessel) is an essential component of colonization, and there is some contrast angiography evidence to support this. However, in some cases, no underlying blood vessel can be demonstrated.

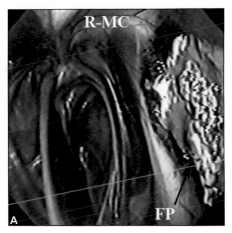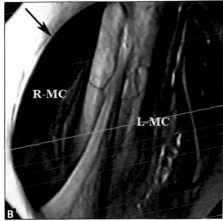

**Figure 4-20A** An endoscopic view of the medial compartment of the right guttural pouch (R-MC) Fungal plaque (FP) involving the medial septum with bilateral extension of lesion.

**Figure 4-20B** An endoscopic view of the medial compartment of the left guttural pouch (L-MC) after successful treatment for the lesion above. Note the complete destruction of the medial septum, with no complications (arrow). Normal architecture of the medial compartment of the contralateral pouch (R-MC) can be viewed via this hole.

Treatment:

✓ The plaque will resolve spontaneously over time and so while not advised – benign neglect may result in remission of the lesion.

✇ Medical therapy using an indwelling catheter (beware significant inflammation results from the placement of these devices) or daily treatment using topical enilconazole 1.7% under endoscopic guidance combined with careful debridement (if lesion is NOT associated with an artery), may result in resolution of infection (Figure 4-21).

♥ Surgical therapy is indicated in cases where there has already been an episode of epistaxis or in cases where the anatomical position of the fungal plaque makes hemorrage highly likely. Intravascular embolization using microcoils or balloon catheters with or without concurrent ligation have been used.

♥ Depending on the position of the fungal plaque, the transverse facial artery, the major palatine artery or the internal carotid artery can be used as entry points for the embolization equipment.

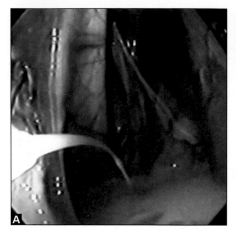
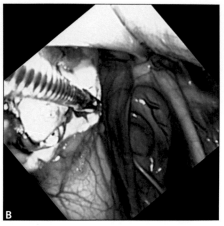

**Figure 4-21A,B** Treatment of guttural pouch mycosis using daily topical lavage using 1.7 % enilconazole (A) via a trans-endoscopic catheter and gentle debridement (B).

# Empyema

✓ Primarily a disease of young foals.

✓ Rupture of the retropharyngeal lymph nodes and drainage into the guttural pouches results in the accumulation of purulent material (Figures 4-22, 4-23, 4-25).

✓ Inflammation in the region of the ventromedial neural plexus can result in severe dysphagia and coughing.

✓ Etiological agents are numerous, however Streptococcus *equi var zooepidemicus* and Strep *equi var equi* remain the most prevalent.

✓ In cases of Strep. *equi var equi* the guttural pouch can remain the source of infectious organisms in clinically normal "carrier animals".

✓ Dehydration of the purulent material sequentially forms thick mucoid pus and then "cottage cheese" consistency, firm and finally hard chondroids (Figure 4-24).

Medical Treatment:

✓ High volume, pressure (>2L/minute with a fluid pump) guttural pouch lavage under sedation.

• Under endoscopic guidance through the endoscope or using an artificial insemination pipette.

💣※ Care should be taken to avoid iatrogenic guttural pouch rupture.

• The use of endoscopic snares to section and remove chondroids.

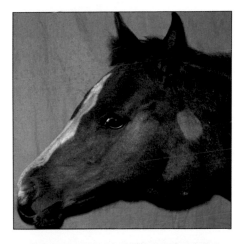

**Figure 4-22** Weanling foal with severe retropharyngeal swelling associated with guttural pouch empyema. Courtesy of Dr. Peter Fretz.

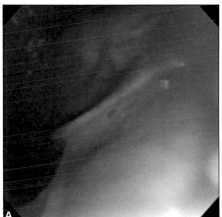
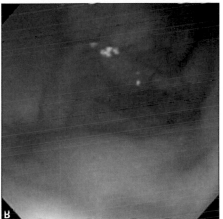

**Figure 4-23A,B** Endoscopic view of the nasopharynx of a foal: Purulent material emanating from the left guttural pouch (A). Endoscopic view of the ventral portion of the medial compartment of the same pouch: Purulent material obscuring the floor (B).

The placement of indwelling catheters

    Catheter placement alone can result in severe inflammation even prior to the addition of therapeutic agents

Systemic antimicrobials

Local infusions

    Mucolytics

      Acetylcysteine-unproven efficacy.

    Antibiotic liquids

      ✓ Antimicrobials held in a gelatin-base may be efficacious.

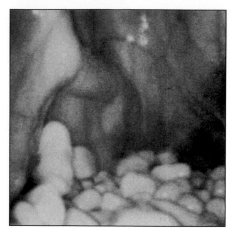

**Figure 4-24** Endoscopic view of the guttural pouch showing pouch showing multiple chondroids on the floor of the medial compartment.
Courtesy of Dr. Peter Fretz

✓ Injection of antimicrobials directly into the offending lymph node via the fistulous tract (Figure 4-25). However this has not been proven to be efficacious.

✓ Treatment can be difficult in chronic cases of empyema as the medial lamina of the guttural pouch opening can become stuck to the axial wall of the nasopharynx (Figure 4-26).

✓ In these cases natural drainage fails to occur.

✓ Re-opening these can present a significant challenge, is time-consuming and painful to the horse.

Surgical Treatment:

✓ There are five different surgical approaches to the guttural pouches (Whitehouse, modified Whitehouse, Viborg's triangle, hyovertebrotomy and Dietrich's approach (a combination of the latter two)).

✓ In cases of chronic disease and poor drainage from the pouch or where chondroids are too large / hard to be removed via the guttural pouch opening.

✓ All surgical options can potentially damage the intra-pouch neural tissue.

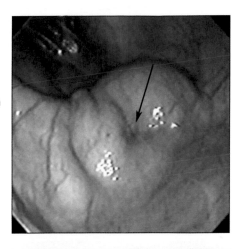

**Figure 4-25** Medial compartment of a right GP (post-flush). Rupture of the retropharyngeal lymph node: Mucus present on floor and fistula (arrow).

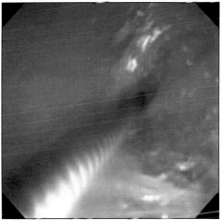

**Figure 4-26** Passage of a biopsy instrument above the plica salpingopharyngea in a case of chronic inflammation. Visibility is poor, hampered by adhesions.

# Temporohyoid Osteoarthropathy

✓ Uncertain etiology but may be the result of trauma to the petrous temporal area, ascending respiratory tract infection, or extension of otitis media or interna.

   ✓ The result is inflammation and fusion of the stylohyoid bone to the petrous temporal bone (Figure 4-27).

   ✓ This may lead to dysfunction of the vestibulocochlear and facial nerves, fracture of the stylohyoid or petrous portion of the temporal bone.

   ✓ Clinical signs can include headshaking, ear flopping and rubbing, signs of vestibular disease, facial paralysis, exposure corneal keratitis (Horner's syndrome) and dysphagia.

   ☙➔ The stylohyoid bone and the temporohyoid articulation should be examined in both pouches.

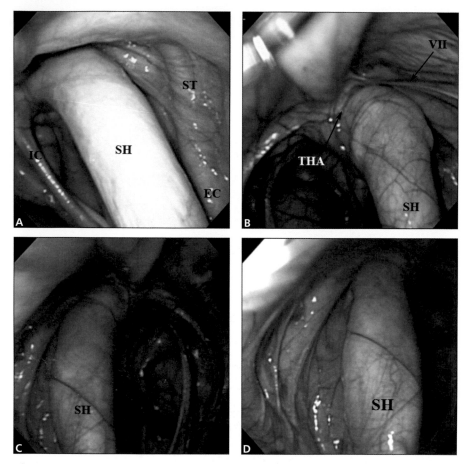

**Figure 4-27A-D** Four different examples of temporohyoid osteoarthropathy. Note differing degress of stylohyoid thickening and temporohyoid thickening, and a clear view of CRN VII (arrow). IC- internal carotid artery, ST – superficial temporal artery, EC – external carotid artery, SH – stylohyoid bone, THA – temporohyoid articulation)

Treatment:

✔ Medical–Antibiotic, anti-inflammatory and corticosteroid therapy.

✔ Surgical–Partial stylohyoidectomy or complete ceratohyoidectomy.

# Inflammation of the Guttural Pouch

Etiology:

✓ Infection–(Bacterial or Fungal)

Iatrogenic:

✓ Use of irritant substances (iodine compounds).

✓ Placement of retention catheters.

Clinical signs:

✓ Range from no obvious abnormalities to dysphagia and coughing.

✓ Mucosal irritation occurs rapidly but can also resolve quickly (Figure 4-28).

✓ Neuritis associated with inflammation may take up to 18 months to resolve.

✓ Some will never resolve entirely.

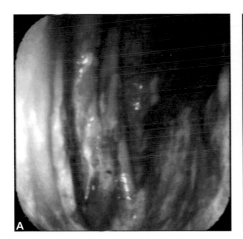 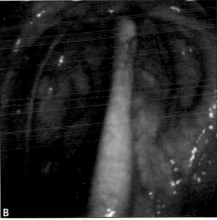

**Figure 4-28A,B** Endoscopic view of the left guttural pouch showing evidence of inflammation. (B) The same guttural pouch after treatment.

# Rupture of the Ventral Straight Muscles of the Neck

✓ Traumatic episode.

✓ Can be accompanied by neurological signs as a compression fracture of the basisphenoid bone can occur.

✓ Can cause severe epistaxis (differential diagnosis: mycosis).

✓ On endoscopic examination of the nasopharynx the roof may be collapsed—usually to a greater degree on the affected side.

✓ Endoscopic examination of the guttural pouch may reveal free hemorrhage within the pouch rostral to the normal arterial structures, in addition to bulging of the medial septum.

✓ Radiographic examination can reveal soft-tissue obliteration of the guttural pouch as well as evidence of basisphenoid fractures.

## Melanomatosis

✓ Common in older grey horses.

✓ Usually an incidental finding as an extension of parotid salivary gland infiltration (Figure 4-29).

✓ No treatment necessary or effective.

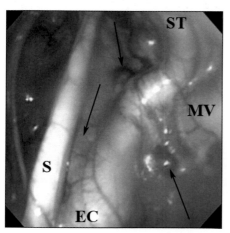

**Figure 4-29** Endoscopic view of the lateral compartment of the left guttural pouch: Note the small black nodular masses (arrows) interspersed across the back of the pouch and the external maxillary artery (EC). ST – superficial temporal artery, MV – maxillary vein, S – stylohyoid bone.
Courtesy of Dr. A. Janzen

## Neoplasia

✓ Squamous cell carcinoma, melanomatosis, round cell sarcoma, hemangioma, hemangiosarcoma, and fibroma have all been reported to occur in the guttural pouch, however these are rare.

# Cysts

✓ Uncertain etiology (congenital or acquired) however they are rare.

# Foreign Bodies

✓ Can include plant material, catheters or wires (Figure 4-30).

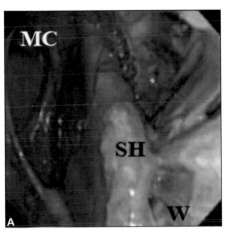

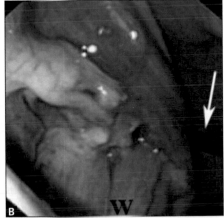

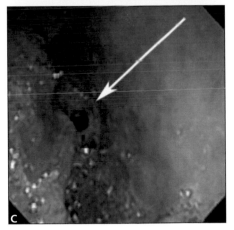

**Figure 4-30A** Endoscopic view of the left guttural pouch. Note the inflammation on the stylohyoid bone (SH), and the presence of a wood (W) foreign body in the lateral compartment. MC – Medial compartment.

**Figure 4-30B** A rostral view of the same pouch, having retroflexed the endoscope (arrow) to examine the rostral extent of the wood (W) and associated mucosal damage.

**Figure 4-30C** An endoscopic view of the caudal aspect of the lateral compartment after wood removal (Figure 4-30A and B) and flushing of the affected pouch. Note the granulation tissue and the continued presence of a small hole (arrow).

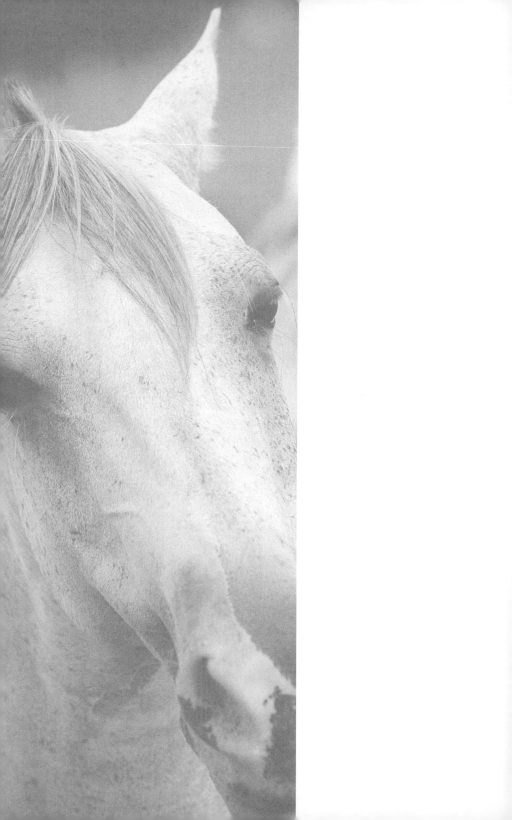

# Section 5

# Endoscopy of the Nasopharynx

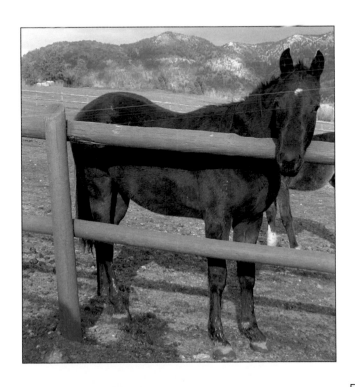

# Anatomy

Tubular structure—Musculomembranous.

Unsupported by cartilage or bone despite tolerating large pressure changes.

The size and shape is altered by a number of intrinsic and extrinsic muscles.

No communication with the oropharynx during normal breathing.

Normal endoscopic structures include the soft palate, guttural pouch openings, dorsal pharyngeal recess, dorsal wall of the nasopharynx, epiglottis and position of the larynx (Figure 5-1).

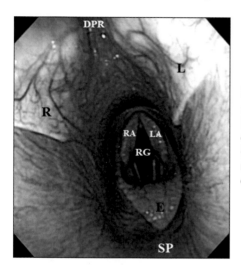

**Figure 5-1** Endoscopic view of a normal nasopharynx in a resting horse. Left (L) and right (R) guttural pouch openings, soft palate (SP), epiglottis (E), rima glottis (RG). Left (LA) and right (RA) arytenoid cartilages and the dorsal pharyngeal recess (DPR).

# Diseases of the Nasopharynx

## Lymphoid Hyperplasia

Aka, pharyngeal hyperplasia, lymphoid follicular hyperplasia.

Inflammation of the pharyngeal lymphoid tissue.

✓ Common in young horses less than 2-3 years old.

✓ Multifactorial etiology but viral (EHV-1 and 2) and secondary bacterial infection and environment play a significant role.

✓ Grading scheme 1-4, with 4 being the most severe (Figure 5-2).

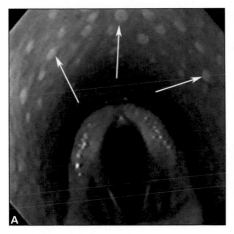 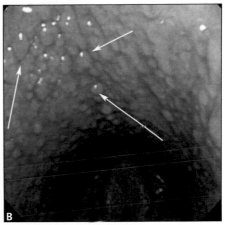

**Figure 5-2A,B** A: Grade 1: Small, white, inactive follicles on dorsal pharyngeal wall (arrows). Normal

B: Grade 2: Many small white follicles, dorsal and lateral walls. Some larger, pink and edematous (arrows)

Grade 3: Many large pink, edematous follicles present on dorsal and lateral walls as well as in dorsal pharyngeal recess +/- soft palate

Strong correlation with age.

Possibly associated with the development of dorsal displacement of the soft palate (DDSP) (Figure 5-4).

Restrict surgical correction until lymphoid hyperplasia resolves and DDSP is proven not to be associated with this inflammatory condition.

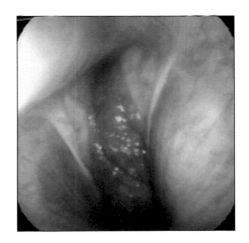

**Figure 5-3** A foal with guttural pouch tympany exhibiting Grade 4 lymphoid follicular hyperplasia: Numerous pink, edematous follicles, coalescing over entire pharynx, epiglottis and mucosal lining of the guttural pouches.

# Dorsal Displacement of the Soft Palate (DDSP)

A condition in which the caudal portion of the soft palate rests above the epiglottis (Figure 5-4).

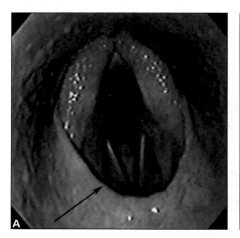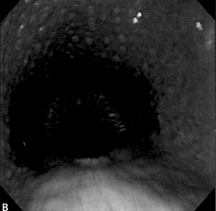

**Figure 5-4A,B** DDSP in two horses. Note the position of the soft palate. The caudal free margin of the soft palate can be visualized, (arrow) the epiglottis cannot.

✓ Two types recognized; Persistent or Intermittent

Persistent

    ✓ Associated with a neuropraxia of the neural input to the soft palate e.g.: guttural pouch inflammation associated with mycosis or empyema. Other causes include true epiglottic abnormalities e.g. : hypoplasia or scarring of the epiglottis following episodes of epiglottitis (Figure 5-5, see Larynx).

    ✓ Clinical signs of the primary disease process predominate in addition to signs of dysphagia (coughing or nasal discharge) (Figure 5-6).

Intermittent

    ♥ Difficult to diagnose during resting endoscopy. It is important _not to sedate the horse_ in order to get an accurate representation of soft palate function.

    ✓ Can perform nasal occlusion test in an attempt to improve likelihood of intermittent DDSP, however this test has a low specificity and sensitivity.

    ✓ Can induce swallowing and attempt to document a failure to replace the soft palate under the epiglottis.

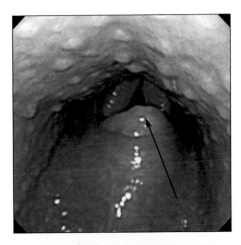

**Figure 5-5** An abnormally short and deformed epiglottis (arrow) causing persistent DDSP in a yearling horse.

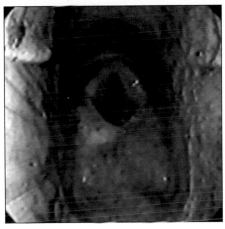

**Figure 5-6** DDSP associated with guttural pouch mycosis. Note the presence of feed material within the nasopharynx.

✓ Treadmill endoscopy is the gold-standard.

Treatment:

Medical:

✓ Management of upper airway inflammation.

✓ Tongue-tie.

✓ Cornell strap.

Surgical:

✓ Staphylectomy- partial soft palate resection.

✓ Myotenectomy of sternothyroideus musculature.

✓ Combination of staphylectomy and myotenectomy.

✓ Oral or per-nasal palatopharyngeoplasty.

✓ Thermal damage to the caudal free margin of the soft palate to induce fibrosis and therefore stiffness of this tissue.

✓ Epiglottic augmentation.

✓ Laryngeal tie-forward.

✓ Laryngeal tie-forward success rate has been reported as 82-87% whereas other methods incur rates of approximately 60%.

# Cleft Palate

Congenital or Iatrogenic.

Congenital (Figure 5-7):

✓ Failure of the palatal folds to close on day 47 of gestation.

✓ Usually, but not always symmetrical in nature.

✓ The folds close in a rostral to caudal direction and thus the disease can involve varying portions of the soft palate or include the hard palate.

✓ Clinical signs typically involve dysphagia, the presence of

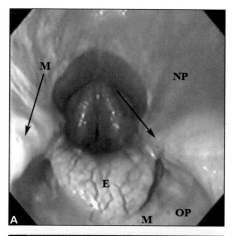
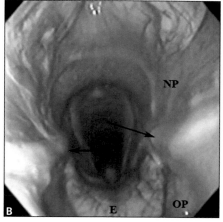
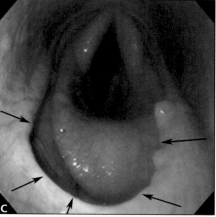

**Figure 5-7A-C** Cleft palate (palatoschisis in a foal): Note the presence of milk in the naso-oro pharynx (M = Milk, NP = Nasopharyx, OP = Oropharynx, E = Epiglottis) Arrows indicate limits of soft palate tissue.

C: Cleft palate in a foal: Note the non-sagittal defect in this case (arrows).

milk at the external nares and coughing.

✓ Aspiration pneumonia is a significant concern and accounts for the majority of the morbidity and mortality associated with this condition.

✓ Surgical correction is possible; however the success rate is approximately 50% for life. No prognosis has been established for racing performance.

Iatrogenic (Figure 5-8):

• Rare, or rarely discussed.

✓ Caused by inaccurate per-nasal axial sectioning of aryepiglottic fold entrapment (See Figure 6-4) using a curved bistory.

✓ The natural equine reaction during this procedure is swallowing.

☞ During the initiation of this maneuver the epiglottis disengages from the soft palate to protect the airway and the soft palate dorsally displaces. This places the caudal free edge of the palate directly under the surgical instrument as it is withdrawn.

✓ The preferred technique is per-oral axial division of the aryepiglottic fold (see section on Endoscopy of the Larynx).

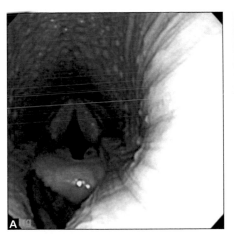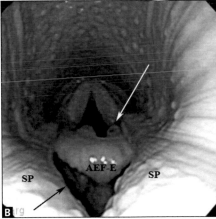

**Figure 5-8A,B** Endoscopic view of a supposed iatrogenic cleft palate.
A: Endoscope placed in the left nostril.
B: Endoscope placed in the right nostril. Note the improved view of the non-sagittal soft palate defect, compared to 5-8A. Attempted resection was likely via this nostril.
Note the presence of the soft palate (SP) as far back as the dorsal pillars, non-sagittal defect, irregular margins of the defect (black arrow) and partial division of the aryepiglottic fold entrapment (AEF-E, white arrow). The horse was euthanased.

# Rostral Displacement of the Palatopharyngeal Arch

✓ Aka, cricopharyngeal-laryngeal dysplasia.

✓ A congenital 4th branchial arch defect characterized by rostral displacement of the ostium intrapharyngeum in addition to abnormally shaped arytenoid cartilages, and absence of cricopharyngeus musculature (Figure 5-9).

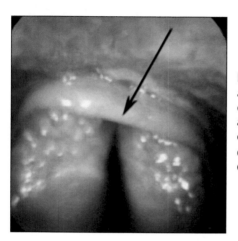

**Figure 5-9** Endoscopic view of the arytenoid cartilages in a case of rostral displacement of the palatopharyngeal arch. Note the rostral placement of the ostium intrapharyngeum (arrow). Courtesy of The Atlantic Veterinary College.

# Collapse of the Dorsal Nasopharynx

✓ Slight collapse occurs in normal horses at the end of expiration due to differential pressures between the nasopharynx and the guttural pouches. In these cases the arytenoid cartilages can still be seen.

✓ Stylopharyngeus muscle dysfunction has been experimentally shown to result in dorsal nasopharynx collapse and theoretically a neuritis could induce this clinical sign (Figure 5-10).

Nasopharyngeal collapse can be static (associated with space-occupying lesions) or dynamic. In the latter case treadmill endoscopy may be necessary to effect a diagnosis.

Clinical signs:

✓ Inspiratory dyspnea and exercise intolerance.

Treatment:

✓ Current therapy revolves around anti-inflammatory treatment as a definitive etiology has not been determined.

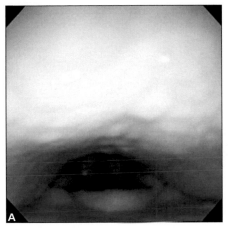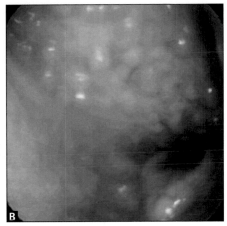

**Figure 5-10A,B** Dorsal collapse of the nasopharynx – Cause undetermined.
A: Dynamic. B: Guttural pouch tympany.

# Choanal Atresia

A bucconasal membrane is present during normal embryological development; this divides the nasal and nasopharyngeal cavities. Failure to resorb this membrane results in choanal atresia (Figure 5-11).

✓ In foals, as in man, the membrane is usually membranous whereas in other species it is primarily bony.

💣 Bilateral cases usually result in foal death.

♥ Unilateral cases present as stertorous breathing and exercise intolerance.

Treatment:

✓ Ablation of the membrane is the goal.

- Sharp dissection using a nasal flap to gain access.
- Sharp dissection using a laryngotomy approach.
- Laser ablation via a videoendoscope.
- Electrosurgical ablation under endoscopic guidance.
- Blunt bougenage (Figure 5-12).

✓ Laser and electrosurgical ablation remains difficult as the membrane is highly vascular which impedes visualization.

✓ Placement of a stent following surgery to prevent reformation of the obstruction is necessary. Despite this re-obstruction is common, even after 4 weeks of stent maintenance.

✓ Prognosis unknown as case numbers are small. However if surgical resection is successful there is no reason why it should not be excellent.

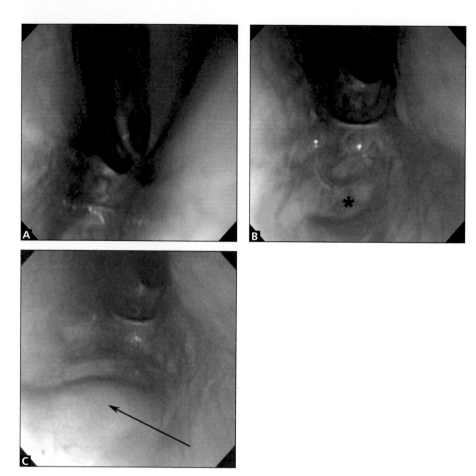

**Figure 5-11A-C** Unilateral right sided choanal atresia in an 8 week old foal.

A: Note position of the ethmoid labyrinth and nasomaxillary opening with no normal opening below it.

B: Ventral view. Entrance to the nasopharynx is blocked (*).

C: Billowing of the structure during expiration – proving it to be membranous (arrow).

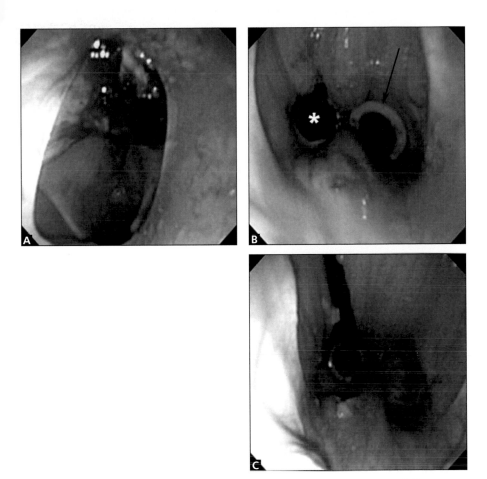

**Figure 5-12A-C** Surgical bougenage of the bucconasal membrane following penetration with a Steinmann pin under general anesthesia (dorsal positioning).

A: Endoscopic view via a 16mm nasotracheal tube.

B: Endoscopic view following retroflexion around the soft palate using an oral approach. The nasopharyngeal tube can be seen in the right nostril (arrow) with the normal nasopharyngeal opening present on the left (*).

C: Same view as above, however endoscope placement via the normal nasopharyngeal opening has occurred with intra-pharyngeal retroflexion.

# Nasopharyngeal Cicatrix

✓ Exclusively seen in hot climates and in horses kept at pasture (Figure 5-13).

✓ Originally reported to occur in older female horses however this has recently been refuted. Age ranges from 5 to 29 have been reported and only 60% are female.

✓ Etiology unknown however an environmental allergen is suspected to cause local inflammation. The resultant scarring reduces the diameter of the nasopharynx.

✓ Most cases have concurrent deformations of epiglottic, arytenoid or guttural pouch osteum cartilage.

✓ Cicatrix formation and position is highly variable.

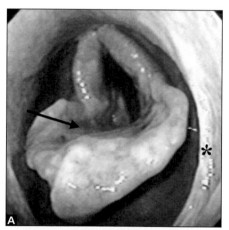

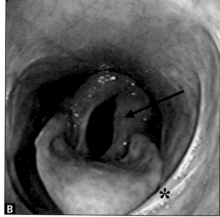

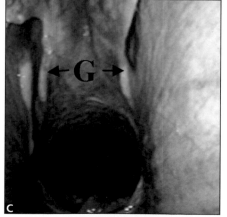

**Figure 5-13A-C** Three different manifestations of nasopharyngeal cicatrix. Note the presence of scar tissue (*), arytenoid abnormalities (arrow) and guttural pouch involvement (G). Courtesy of Dr. Jim Schumacher.

# Nasopharyngeal Masses

Rare.

✓ As with masses of the nasal passages those of the nasopharynx are usually extensions of sinus, oropharynx or guttural pouch disease (see epiglottic cysts).

✓ Fungal granulomas, cysts and neoplastic processes such as squamous cell carcinoma and lymphosarcoma have been reported as primary disease.

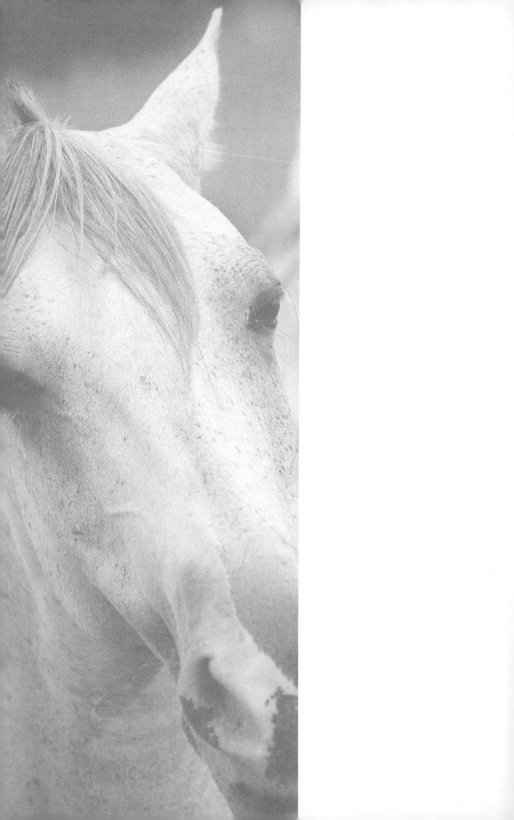

# Section 6

# Endoscopy of the Larynx

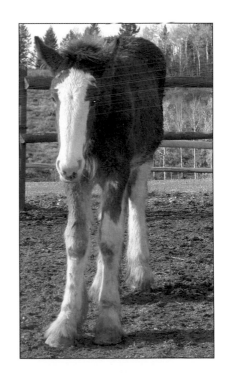

# Anatomy

✓ Composed unpaired cricoid, thyroid and epiglottic cartilages as well as paired arytenoid cartilages and vocal chords (Figure 6-1).

✓ Joins the pharynx and the trachea.

✓ Intrinsic musculature alters the diameter of the rima glottis.

✓ Mucosa of the larynx is tightly adherent to the underlying cartilages other than under the epiglottis where it is loosely attached.

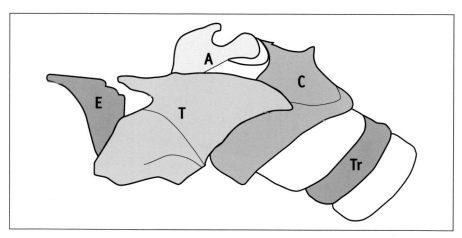

**Figure 6-1A** Lateral anatomical view of the larynx showing the epiglottis (E), thyroid (T), cricoid (C) and arytenoid (A) cartilages as well as the first tracheal ring (Tr).

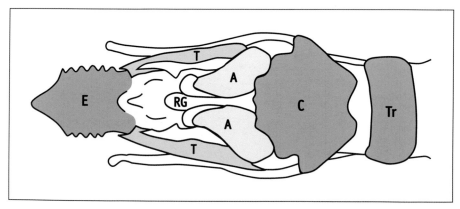

**Figure 6-1B** Dorsal anatomical view of the larynx showing the epiglottis (E), thyroid laminae (T), cricoid (C), paired arytenoid cartilages (A), rima glottis (RG) and first tracheal ring (Tr).

# Endoscopic Technique

Place endoscope in ventral meatus of nose and advance it until the tip is in the middle of the soft palate. The entire larynx should be visualized from this position (Figures 6-2 and 6-3).

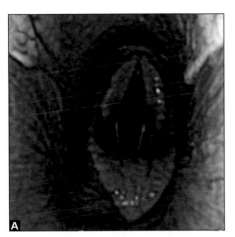
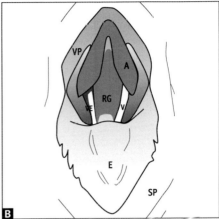

**Figure 6-2A,B** A normal endoscopic view and artist's rendition of the rima glottis (RG), arytenoid cartilages (A), vocal cords (V) and ventricles (VE), epiglottis (E), rostral soft palate position (SP) and vertical pillars of the soft palate (VP).

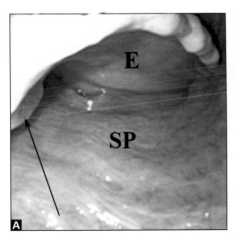
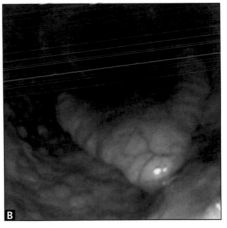

**Figure 6-3A,B** A: Endoscopic view of the floor of the nasopharynx, immediately below the epiglottic tip. Note the curled nature of the tip (arrow) and the more vertical position of the epiglottis (E) above the soft palate (SP). A version of normal

B: Endoscopic view of the caudal nasopharynx. Note the pointed and flattened nature of the epiglottis. A version of normal.

# Diseases of the Larynx

## Aryepiglottic Fold Entrapment

✓ Aka epiglottic entrapment.

✓ Loose ventral mucosa become trapped over the rostral free edge of the epiglottis.

✓ Endoscopically the epiglottis is still visible above the margin of the soft palate however; the normal crenellated edge and dorsal vasculature of the cartilage are obscured (Figure 6-4).

✓ Entrapping mucosa can be thick or thin, narrow or wide and ulcerated or not. Most are thick, wide and ulcerated.

✓ Some degree of hypoplasia of the epiglottis is common with this disease.

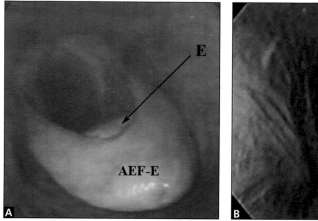
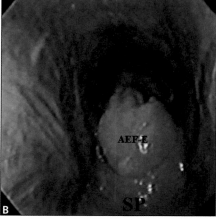

**Figure 6-4A,B** Aryepiglottic fold entrapment: Note the smooth, rounded tissue in the epiglottic region (AEF-E), the normal position of the soft palate (SP) and the epiglottis behind the tissue (E, arrow).

✓ Axial division of the mucosal tissue is the treatment of choice.

✓ Transendoscopic laser, per-nasal or per oral division using a curved bistory, or division via a laryngotomy or pharyngotomy incision (Figure 6-5).

💣 **Note:** Axial division per-nasum is to be avoided due to the distinct risk of the iatrogenic creation of a cleft palate (See Figure 5-8).

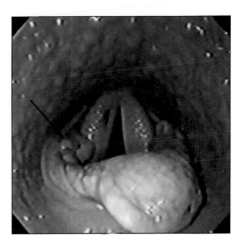

**Figure 6-5** Post-surgical view of the epiglottis following axial sectioning of the entrapping tissue via a pharyngotomy incision. Note the presence of persistent tissue on the right of the epiglottis (arrow) which was subsequently removed.

# Axial Deviation of the Aryepiglottic Folds

✓ Occurs during maximal exertion and is therefore a diagnosis based on treadmill examination and not resting endoscopy.

✓ Results in inspiratory dyspnea, noise and exercise intolerance.

✓ Bilateral involvement is most commonly reported, however right-sided uni-axial deviation has been diagnosed.

# Epiglottic Retroversion

✓ Etiology unknown, however based on experimental work a neuritis or neuralgia of the hypoglossal nerve or the geniohyoid muscle is likely.

✓ Endoscopy at rest is unlikely to render a diagnosis as the nasopharynx is either normal or the epiglottis sits just slightly above the level of the soft palate which may be misconstrued as a version of normal (See Figure 6-3).

✓ Treadmill endoscopy can reveal intermittent abnormalities in the positioning of this structure with concurrent occlusion of the rima glottis (Figure 6-6).

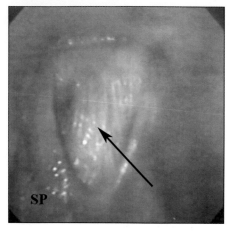

**Figure 6-6** Epiglottic Retroversion: Endoscopic view of the caudal portion of the soft palate (SP) showing the underside of the epiglottis and the hyoepiglotticus muscle (arrow).

# Epiglottitis

✓ Etiology unknown.

✓ Most commonly seen in Thoroughbred racehorses.

✓ Epiglottis appears thickened, edematous and may be reddened.

✓ Swelling may elevate the epiglottis into an abnormal position within the nasopharynx.

✓ Anti-inflammatory therapy is the treatment of choice.

✓ Up to 50% of the horses will incur long term complications including epiglottic malformation, entrapment or dorsal displacement of the soft palate (Figure 6-7).

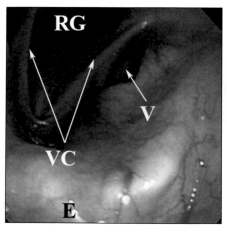

**Figure 6-7** A pharyngoscopic (via the mouth) view of the epiglottis in a horse under general anesthesia in which epiglottic deformity (presumably following an episode of epiglottitis – as the foal had been born and developed normally) had resulted in permanent DDSP (See Nasopharynx section, Figure 5-5). Note the thickened and abaxial placement of the epiglottis (E). The ventral aspect of the rima glottis (RG), vocal chords (VC) and left ventricle (V) can be seen.

# Subepiglottic Cysts

Remnant of the embryological thyroglossal duct.

✓ Can be congenital or in some cases acquired as they can be found in older horses with no previous history of upper airway problems.

✓ Clinical signs can include coughing, noise or dysphagia (Figure 6-8).

Treatment:

✓ Surgical ablation of the mass – simple drainage will result in refilling of the cyst.

• Laryngotomy or per-oral approaches using sharp or laser dissection.

• Removal using embryotomy wire via a per-oral approach has also been successful (Figure 6-9).

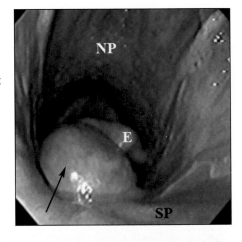

**Figure 6-8** A large sub-epiglottic cyst (arrow), below the epiglottis (E). While the horse presented with intermittent DDSP and coughing, in this view the soft palate (SP) is in the normal position. (NP – Nasopharynx) .

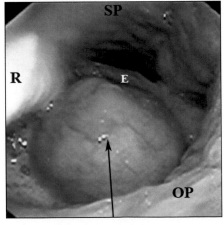

**Figure 6-9** Intra-operative pharyngoscopic (OP- oropharynx) view of the sub-epiglottic cyst (arrow) seen above (Figure 6-8). The rod (R) was comprised of two artificial insemination pipettes taped together enclosing a loop of Gigli wire. (E-epiglottis, SP – Soft palate).

↧ It is important not to remove too much of the loose sub-epiglottic tissue during extirpation of the cyst as scar formation below the epiglottis may interfere with its' shape and function (Figure 6-10).

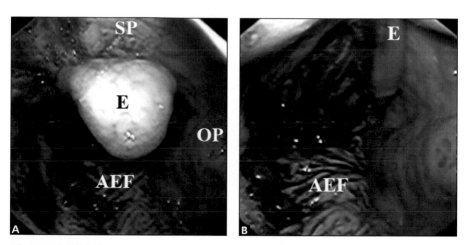

**Figure 6-10A,B** Post-operative pharyngoscopic (OP – oropharynx) view of the sub-epiglottic cyst (Figure 6-8). The epiglottic tip (E) has retained the normal curved shape (A), the cyst has been completely removed and the amount of remaining loose sub-epiglottic mucosal tissue (AEF) was sufficient to prevent cicatrix formation (B).

# Arytenoid Chondritis

A septic inflammation of the arytenoid cartilage.

Produces axial deviation of the cartilage and respiratory noise.

✓ Classical endoscopic signs include swelling of the affected arytenoid cartilage, the presence of a draining tract or granulomatous tissue and arytenoid distortion (Figures 6-11 and 6-12).

Care:

✓ This may mimic laryngeal hemiplegia due to the abnormal position, especially if the other classical signs (above) are not present.

✓ Acute presentations with horses in respiratory distress can occur due to laryngeal edema and these cases may require an emergency tracheotomy.

Treatment:

• Most cases respond well to anti-inflammatory (systemic and/or topical) and antimicrobial therapy.

**Figure 6-11** Arytenoid chondritis of the right arytenoid of a mature horse. Note the swollen arytenoid (black arrow) and presence of a draining tract in the mid-laminar portion of the cartilage (white arrow).

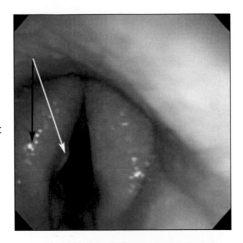

**Figure 6-12** An endoscopic view of the larynx of a mature horse that presented with coughing and dyspnea. Note the presence of uniaxial left sided edema and reddening of the tissue. This was an early case of arytenoid chondritis.

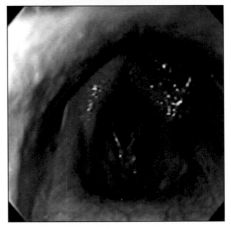

- Arytenoid cartilage deformation may remain following treatment. If the deformation does not impede airway function the cartilage can perform well (Figure 6-13).

✔ If medical therapy fails to resolve the chondritis or residual deformation results in laryngeal obstruction, surgical ablation of the affected tissue may be necessary. Using sharp or laser debridement of the infected tissue, or removal of the affected arytenoid.

✔ A partial arytenoidectomy combined with a ventriculocordectomy results in a better success rate than a subtotal arytenoidectomy.

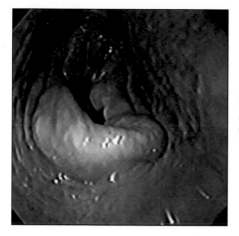

**Figure 6-13** Arytenoid cartilage and aryepiglottic fold malformation following chronic arytenoid chondritis.

# Left Laryngeal Hemiplegia

✓ Associated with a loss of long myelinated fibers within the recurrent laryngeal nerve leading to neurogenic atrophy of the intrinsic musculature of the larynx, most notably the cricoarytenoideus dorsalis muscle.

✓ Adductor function fails first (rarely appreciated) followed by the more readily identified failure in abductor function.

✓ Graded from 1 (Normal) to 4 (complete failure to abduct during inspiration and in some cases pulled across the midline of the rima glottis by negative inspiratory pressure) (Figure 6-14, Table 6-1).

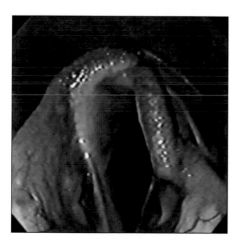

**Figure 6-14** A Grade 4 left laryngeal hemiplegia.

## Table 6-1
## Subjective Grading of Laryngeal Movement in Horses with Suspected Laryngeal Hemiplegia
Adapted from Auer and Stick, 2006

| GRADE | MOVEMENT |
|-------|----------|
| 1 | Symmetrical, synchronous movement of both arytenoid cartilages during inspiration and expiration. |
| 2 | Slight asynchrony in movement between left and right cartilages. Full abduction can still be attained during swallowing, nasal occlusion or treadmill endoscopy. |
| 3 | Asynchronous movement of cartilages during abduction and adduction. Full abduction may (Grade 3A) or may not (Grade 3B) be attained during maximal exercise. |
| 4 | No significant movement during respiration. Affected cartilage hangs in midline and on inspiration, especially under strenuous conditions, moves across midline in response to negative pressures within airway. |

Treatment:

- Laryngoplasty (tie-back) (Figure 6-15).
- Ventriculectomy (sacculectomy).
- Ventriculocordectomy.
- Partial arytenoidectomy.
- Combined laryngoplasty / ventriculocordectomy.
- Neuromuscular pedicle graft.

✓ If NOISE is the primary problem (e.g.: showhorses) a bilateral ventriculocordectomy should be performed. However this procedure will only realize a limited improvement in airflow dynamics.

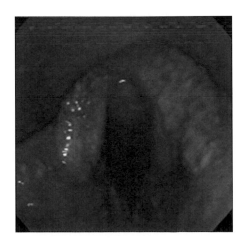

**Figure 6-15** Endoscopic view of the arytenoid cartilages following laryngoplasty the previous day. Note the left cartilage in an abducted position but not pulled too far laterally in an effort to reduce the incidence of post-operative coughing.

✓ If _PERFORMANCE_ (speed) is the primary problem, air flow dynamics are improved maximally by performing a laryngoplasty rather than a ventriculochordectomy.

✓ There is no reported benefit to racing performance of combining a laryngoplasty with uniaxial ventriculochordectomy.

⚷➔ Complications of laryngoplasty can include coughing and initial signs of discomfort during eating (as protection of the upper airway during swallowing is compromised) as well as failure of the fixation (cartilage failure or suture failure).

# Right Laryngeal Hemiplegia

Rare.

✓ Congenital malformation or acquired via an associated neuritis (such as a guttural pouch disease).

Prognosis is good if the underlying neuritis can be treated successfully (See endoscopy of the guttural pouch). Prognosis is poor if associated with congenital malformation of the arytenoid cartilages.

# Biaxial Laryngeal Hemiplegia

Rare

Etiology:

- Organophosphate toxicity.
- Systemic diseases such as equine protozoal meningoencephalitis (EPM) or hepatic disease.
- A rare complication of inhalation anesthesia.

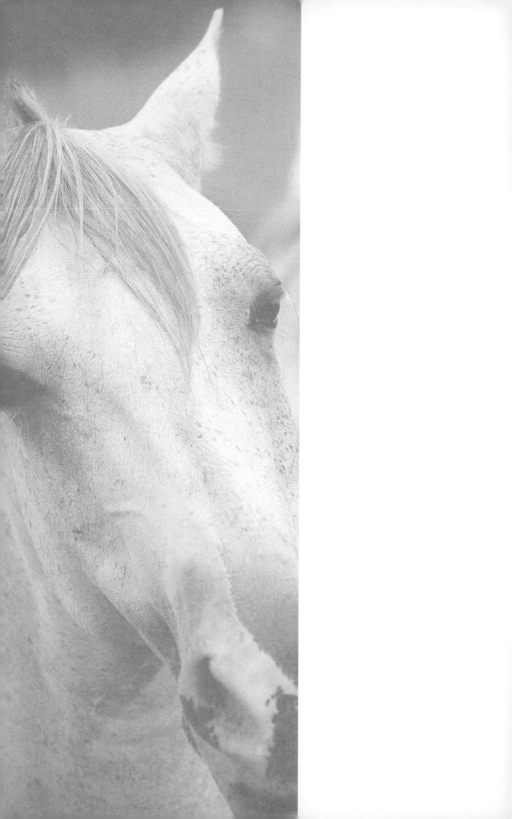

# Section 7

# Endoscopy of the Trachea and Bronchi

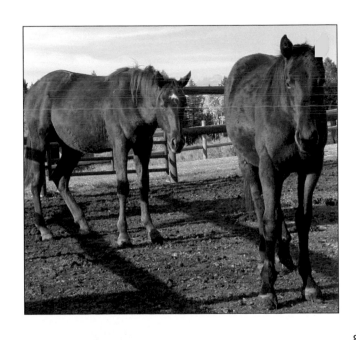

# Anatomy

The trachea is a cylindrical tube that extends from the larynx to the lungs.

It is non-collapsible and formed by a series of adjacent cartilage rings, which are incomplete dorsally.

✓ The trachea is about 80 cm in length and has a diameter of 5-7 cm, depending on the size of the horse.

It is circular in shape, especially at the origin and in the thoracic area.

✓ However, the lumen of the trachea may appear dorsoventrally flattened in the cervical area and this varies with the phase of respiration (inspiration vs expiration).

The trachea terminates and branches into two main stem bronchi, one for each lung, at the level of the base of the heart.

The main stem bronchi branch into smaller bronchi and finally form smaller branches called bronchioles.

# Endoscopic Technique and Normal Endoscopic Findings

✓ Endoscopic examination of the trachea is usually performed in the standing, conscious horse, however sedation may be needed.

✓ The recommended length of the endoscope used is about 150 cm.

✓ The tip of the endoscope is passed through the ventral meatus of the nose to the naso-pharynx and positioned in the center, just in front of the arytenoids (Figure 7-1).

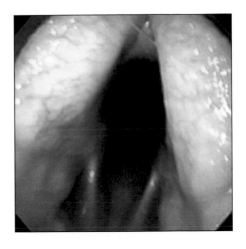

**Figure 7-1** The tip of the endoscope should be positioned in the center of the rima glottis, just in front of the arytenoids, before it is passed into the trachea.

✓ Once the arytenoids are abducted, the tip of the endoscope should be passed into the trachea (Figure 7-2).

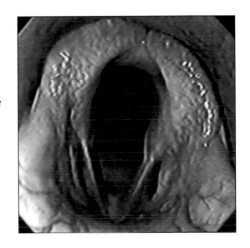

**Figure 7-2** The tip of the endoscope should be passed into the trachea after the arytenoids are abducted (on inspiration).

✓ The normal tracheal mucosa ranges between pale yellow to pale pink in color.

The tracheal lining is smooth with visible vasculature. The tracheal rings are detectable (Figure 7-3).

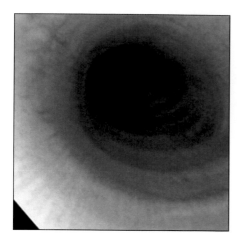

**Figure 7-3** Normal tracheal mucosa. Note the smooth tracheal lining with visible vasculature and tracheal rings.

✓ The trachea is normally free of exudate or discharge.

✓ The carina, principal and lobar bronchi are seen at the most distal part of the trachea (Figure 7-4).

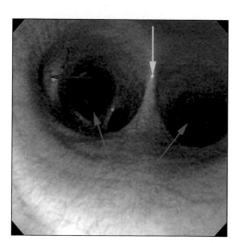

**Figure 7-4** The most distal part of the trachea. The carina (yellow arrow). Principal (blue arrows) and lobar bronchi (red arrow).

# Diseases of the Trachea

## Tracheal Collapse

✓ It is deemed to be congenital.

It is usually seen in ponies and miniature horses.

✓ Abnormal breathing sounds may be heard.

Endoscopy of the trachea reveals a collapsed and narrowed lumen (Figure 7-5).

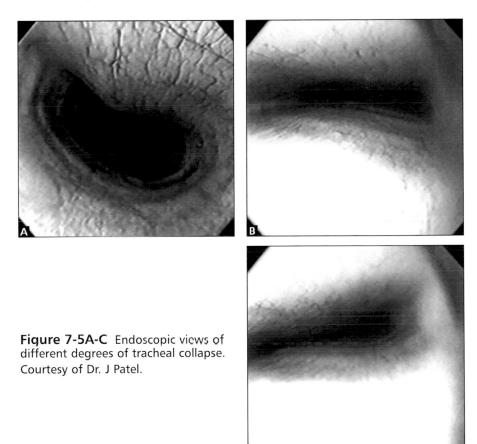

**Figure 7-5A-C** Endoscopic views of different degrees of tracheal collapse. Courtesy of Dr. J Patel.

# Tracheitis

✓ Usually caused by viral infection of the upper respiratory tract.

✓ The tracheal mucosa is usually red in color and may look roughened.

There may be mucopurulant material adhered to the tracheal mucosa (Figure 7-6).

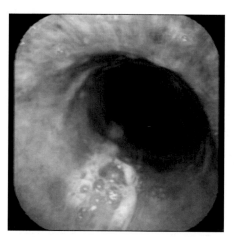

**Figure 7-6** The tracheal mucosa is red and roughened in a horse with tracheitis. Note the mucopurulant material that is adhered to the tracheal mucosa. Courtesy of the Atlantic Veterinary College.

# Tracheal Luminal Obstruction and Masses

Causes:

✓ Neoplasia such as squamous cell carcinoma

✓ Fibrotic stricture following trauma.

✓ Foreign bodies such as food or sand (after racing).

✓ Compression from an extra luminal mass such as an abscess or neoplasm.

✓ Fungal granuloma.

✓ Granulation tissue.

✓ Chondroma as a sequela to trans-tracheal punctures.

# Miscellaneous Conditions

Tracheal rupture or fistula may be seen secondary to trauma.

# Gross Tracheal Discharge

Blood:

- Causes include exercise-induced pulmonary hemorrhage (EIPH)
  - ✓ EIPH is usually categorized on a scale of 0-4 (1 hour post-exercise) (Figure 7-7 through 7-11).

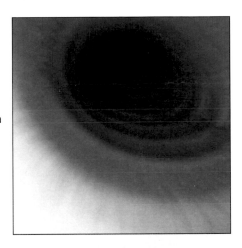

**Figure 7-7** EIPH Score 0 : No blood is detected in the pharynx, larynx, trachea or main stem bronchi. Courtesy of Dr. L. Couetil, Purdue University.

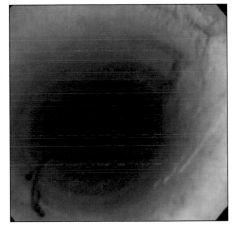

**Figure 7-8** EIPH Score 1: Presence of 1 or more flecks of blood or 2 or fewer short (<1/4 length of the trachea), narrow (<10% of the tracheal surface area) streams of blood in the trachea or main stem bronchi visible from the tracheal bifurcation. Courtesy of Dr. L. Couetil, Purdue University

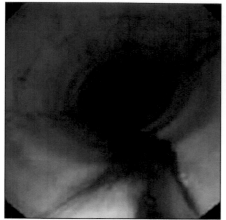

**Figure 7-9** EIPH Score 2: one long stream of blood (greater than half the length of the trachea) or more than 2 short streams of blood are occupying less than a third of the tracheal circumference. Courtesy of Dr. L. Couetil, Purdue University.

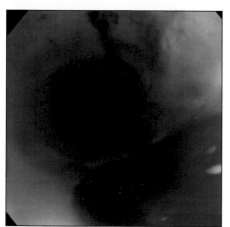

**Figure 7-10** EIPH Score 3: Multiple, distinct streams of blood covering more than 1/3 of the tracheal circumference, with no blood pooling at the thoracic inlet. Courtesy of Dr. L. Couetil, Purdue University.

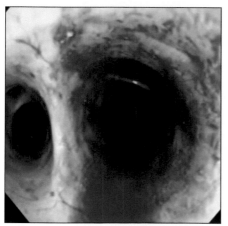

**Figure 7-11** EIPH Score 4: Multiple, coalescing streams of blood covering >90 % of the tracheal surface, with blood pooling at the thoracic inlet. Courtesy of Dr. L. Couetil, Purdue University.

✔ Occasionally, blood may be found in the trachea of horses with guttural pouch mycosis, due to dysphagia (Figure 7-12).

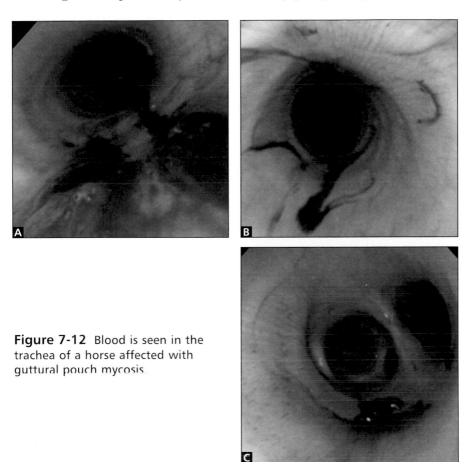

**Figure 7-12** Blood is seen in the trachea of a horse affected with guttural pouch mycosis.

Mucus / Mucopurulent discharge / Pus:

✔ Creamy, yellow or pale white in color.

• Causes include recurrent airway obstruction (previously known as COPD (Figure 7-13).

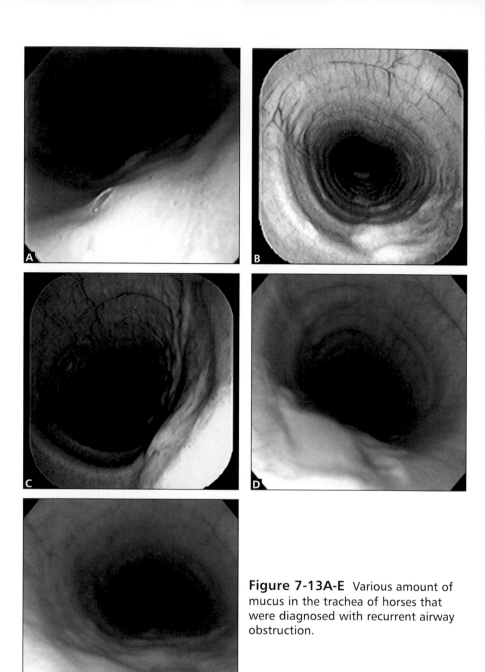

**Figure 7-13A-E** Various amount of mucus in the trachea of horses that were diagnosed with recurrent airway obstruction.

✓ Lower air way infection or inflammation caused by *Streptococcus zooepidemicus* (Figure 7-14).

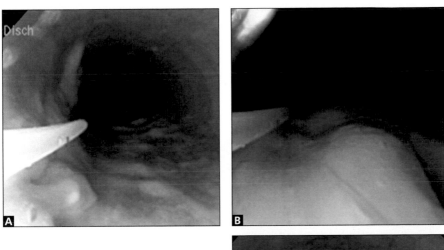

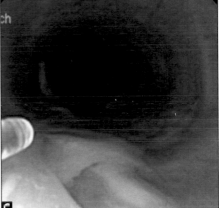

**Figure 7-14A-C** Mucopurulent tracheal discharge is usually seen in horses with lower air way infection caused by *Streptococcus zooepidemicus.*

- Allergic upper air way inflammation (Figure 7-15).

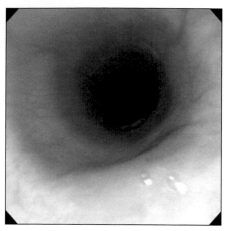

**Figure 7-15** Mucus can be seen in horses with allergic upper air way inflammation. This endoscopic view was obtained from a horse with signs of peracute upper air way inflammation, edema and anaphylaxis.

- Severe pneumonia may be associated with the presence of yellow-brown colored mucus (Figure 7-16).

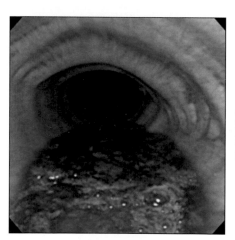

**Figure 7-16** Yellow-brown colored mucus can be seen in the trachea of horses with severe pneumonia. This horse had pneumonia caused by a mixed bacterial infection.

- Pus may be seen in the trachea of horses with lung abscesses (Figure 7-17).

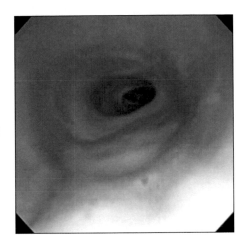

**Figure 7-17** Endoscopic view of the trachea in a foal affected with lung abscesses. Note the pus in the tracheal lumen.

Food / Milk / Saliva:

✓ It is usually seen in the trachea of horses with dysphagia.

# Tracheal Wash and Aspirate

Tracheal wash can be performed using the endoscope or percutaneously.

✓ The endoscope allows the examiner to visualize the airways as well as the fluid sample that is being collected.

✓ In addition, endoscopy is associated with fewer complications, when compared with the percutaneous transtracheal wash method.

✓ The horse should be restrained. Sedation may not be required.

✓ The tip of the endoscope is passed into the trachea in a routine fashion.

✓ Fluid or discharge in the trachea usually forms a pool at the level of the thoracic inlet (Figure 7-18).

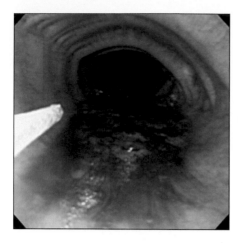

**Figure 7-18** Fluid or discharge in the trachea usually forms a pool at the level of the thoracic inlet.

A guarded or double sheath catheter is usually used to avoid contamination of the collected sample by the equipment (endoscopy channel) (Figure 7-19).

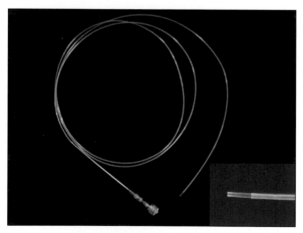

**Figure 7-19** A guarded or double sheath catheter.

A guarded or double sheath catheter is passed through the biopsy channel. Once the tip of the catheter is visualized, the operator should advance the inside catheter.

20-40 ml of sterile, isotonic saline is infused and immediately aspirated from the airway. Aspiration of the fluid is usually aimed at the pool which is at the thoracic inlet (Figures 7-20 and 7-21).

After the sample is collected, the catheter is withdrawn followed by the endoscope.

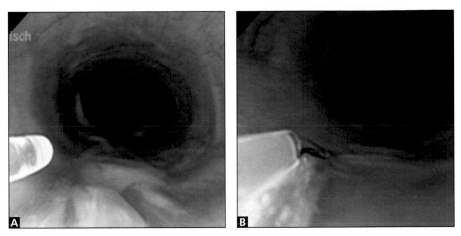

**Figure 7-20A,B** After the guarded or double sheath catheter is passed through the biopsy channel and once the tip of the catheter is visualized. The operator should advance the inside catheter and infuse the isotonic saline as seen in the above endoscopic views.

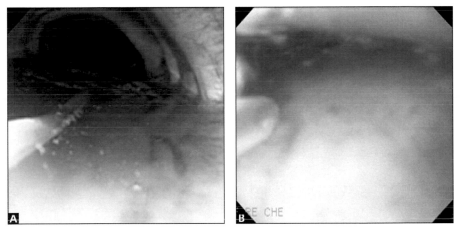

**Figure 7-21A,B** After the isotonic saline is infused it should be immediately aspirated from the trachea. The operator can visualize the tip of the endoscope and make sure that the tip is always immersed in the fluid pool during aspiration of the fluid.

# Bronchioalveolar Lavage

✔ Bronchioalveolar lavage can be performed using the endoscope, or a special catheter, which is passed intranasaly.

Using the endoscope will allow visualization of the airways.

✔ An endoscope at least 180-200 cm long is recommended.

The horse should be restrained and sedated.

✔ The biopsy channel should be cleaned using antiseptic solution and rinsed with sterile water.

The tip of the endoscope is passed into the trachea in a routine fashion. It should be advanced further until the tip of the endoscope is wedged in a bronchus, to facilitate suction of the infused fluids (Figures 7-22 and 7-23).

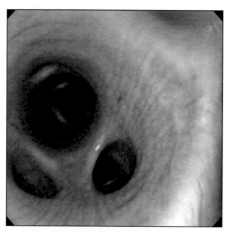

**Figure 7-22**  The tip of the endoscope should be passed through the bronchial tree until the tip of the endoscope is wedged in a bronchus.

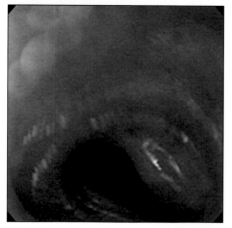

**Figure 7-23**  View with the tip of the endoscope wedged in a bronchus.

✎ If the horse starts to cough excessively, 20-40 ml of 2% lidocaine may be infused in to the airways using the biopsy channel.

✓ 100-300 ml of warm, isotonic saline may be infused through the biopsy channel and aspirated immediately using a vacuum suction.

✓ 50-80 % of the infused volume is usually retrieved and is foamy in nature.

✓ Once the sample is collected, the endoscope is withdrawn.

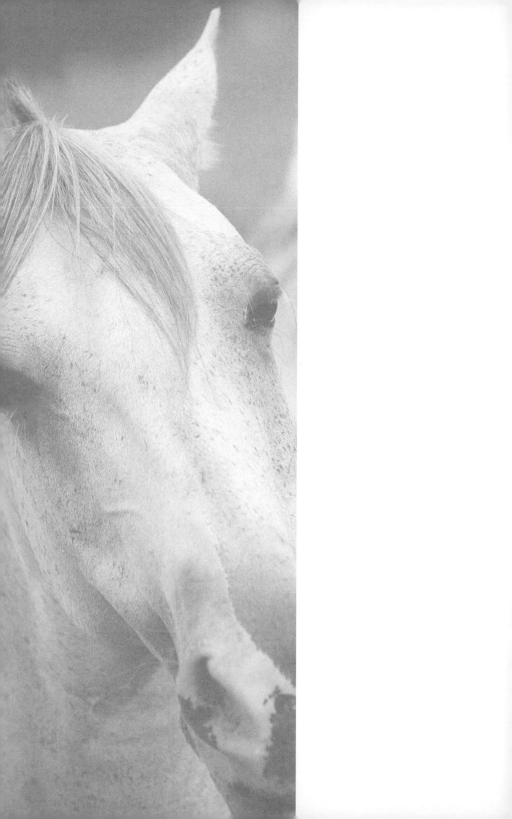

# Section 8
# Endoscopy of the Esophagus

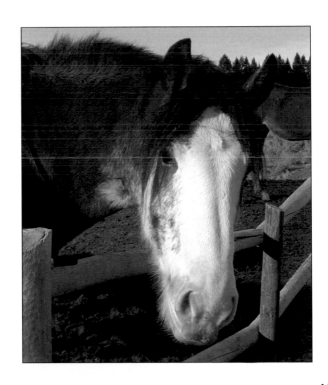

# Anatomy

The esophagus is a tubular structure that is about 120 cm in length (500 kg horse).

It is divided into three parts; cervical, thoracic and abdominal.

In the cervical region, the esophagus lies dorsal and slightly to the left of the trachea.

✔ The proximal two thirds of the esophagus contains striated muscles while the distal third contains smooth muscle.

The esophagus has an upper and lower sphincters:

✔ The upper sphincter is encountered after the pharyngeal-esophageal junction (Figure 8-1).

✔ The lower sphincter terminates the esophagus and enters the cardia of the stomach (Figure 8-2).

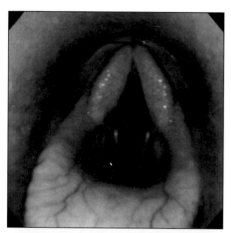

**Figure 8-1** The upper esophageal sphincter is encountered after the pharyngeal-esophageal junction (arrow). The tip of the scope is aimed dorsal to the arytenoid cartilages (arrow).

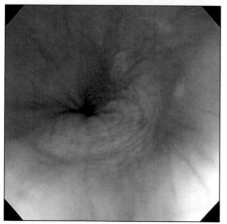

**Figure 8-2** The lower esophageal sphincter.

# Endoscopic Technique

✓ The animal should be properly restrained or sedated.

✓ The endoscope is advanced through the ventral meatus to the nasopharynx in a manner similar to the passage of a nasogastric tube.

✓ The esophageal opening lies dorsal to the arytenoid cartilages and slightly on the left side.

Once the endoscope is advanced to the pharynx, the tip is aimed dorsal to the arytenoid cartilages (Figure 8-1), then advanced to the upper esophageal sphincter.

✓ The passage of the endoscope is facilitated by stimulating the swallowing reflex.

✓ The swallowing reflex can be stimulated by repeated touching of the area dorsal to the arytenoid cartilages using the tip of the endoscope, or by spraying a small amount of water using the water source.

Further advancement of the endoscope should follow the swallowing act.

✓ If the horse is sedated, the swallowing reflex might be depressed or slow.

Do not keep advancing the endoscope in the esophagus unless it is confirmed that the endoscope is in the right path and not retroflexed.

☛ Retroflexion may advance the endoscope to the mouth where the endoscope might get severely damaged (chewed off).

If the endoscope or teeth are seen, the endoscope should be withdrawn immediately until the right path is identified (Figures 8-3 and 8-4).

The esophagus should be examined while passing the endoscope. However, examining the esophagus during withdrawal, while the esophagus is insufflated may provide a better view (Figure 8-5).

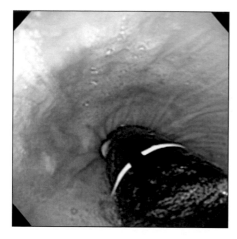

**Figure 8-3** Retroflexion of the endoscope in the esophagus.

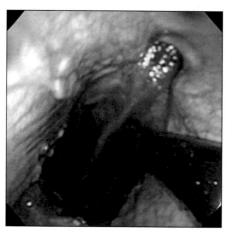

**Figure 8-4** Retroflexion in the pharynx may advance the endoscope to the mouth and cause subsequent damage to the endoscope. Nasal septum (arrow).

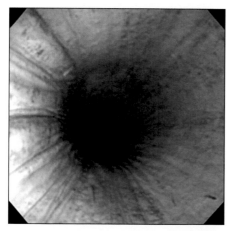

**Figure 8-5** Viewing the esophagus during withdrawal while insufflated.

# Normal Endoscopic Findings

The mucosa of the esophagus is glistening, whitish gray or pink and has longitudinal folds. If examined while collapsed, the esophagus may also have temporary transverse folds (Figure 8-6).

✓ A small amount of saliva containing air bubbles may be seen in the normal esophagus, but this should be cleared quickly by peristaltic movement.

The lower esophageal sphincter is usually closed (Figure 8-7).

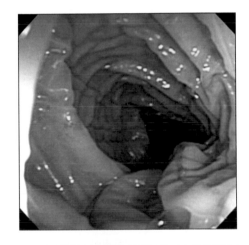

**Figure 8-6** Esophageal folds.

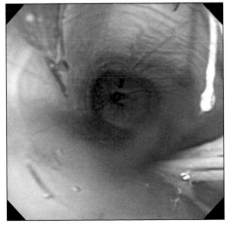

**Figure 8-7** Closed lower esophageal sphincter.

# Diseases of the Esophagus

## Esophageal Obstruction (Choke)

Choke is defined as obstruction of the lumen of the esophagus. Choke is the most common esophageal disorder that is seen in horses.

✓ It can be partial or complete and either primary (simple choke) or secondary to other disease processes.

## A-Primary choke:

✓ Caused by feed, particularly leafy alfalfa, coarse grass hay, grass, improperly soaked sugar beet, or foreign bodies (e.g. stones, bedding, medicinal boluses, carrot, apple, corncobs, potato, wood fragments).

✓ It is more common in old horses.

• There are four common anatomical areas of natural narrowing in the esophagus, where primary choke usually occurs. These include the post pharyngeal area, thoracic inlet, base of the heart, and close to the cardia of the stomach (terminal esophagus) (Figure 8-8).

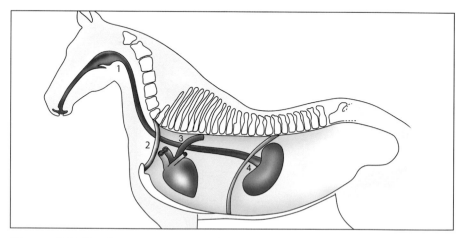

**Figure 8-8** The four common areas for primary choke.1- post pharyngeal area, 2- thoracic inlet, 3- base of the heart, and 4- close to the cardia of the stomach. Drawing by Dr. Juliane Deubner

Clinical signs are usually acute in nature and include anxiety, standing with the head and neck extended, gagging or retching, painful repeated attempts at swallowing, bilateral frothy nasal discharge containing feed material and saliva, coughing and drooling of saliva (Figures 8-9 and 8-10).

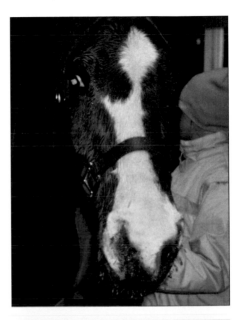

**Figure 8-9** Bilateral nasal discharge containing feed material in a horse with choke.

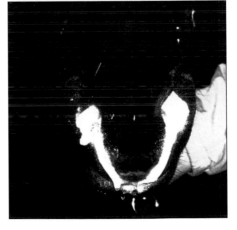

**Figure 8-10** Bilateral white, frothy nasal discharge in a horse with choke.

✓ If the cervical esophagus is ruptured or perforated, swelling (cellulitis) and crepitus may result (Figure 8-11).

♥ If the obstruction is in the cervical area of the esophagus, or causes feed accumulation in the cervical esophagus, a palpable or visible mass on the left lateroventral aspect of the neck may be felt.

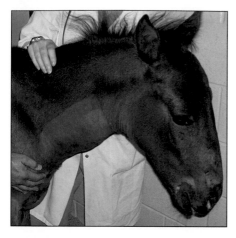

**Figure 8-11** Esophageal perforation in a foal with esophageal obstruction caused by a foreign body. Note the neck swelling due to cellulitis.

Endoscopic findings in primary esophageal obstruction:

• Endoscopic examination of the esophagus is very helpful in the diagnosis and treatment of esophageal obstruction.

✓ A one to two meter endoscope should be used; the required length depends on the site of obstruction and the size of the horse.

• In large horses even a two meter endoscope may not reach the cardia of the stomach.

• When the endoscope is passed to the pharynx, feed or white foam may be seen in cases of esophageal obstruction (Figures 8-12 and 8-13).

• Sometimes, white foam will overflow from the esophagus (Figure 8-14).

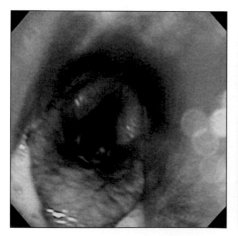
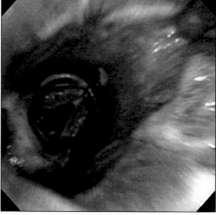

**Figures 8-12 and 8-13** White foam in the nasopharynx of a horse with esophageal obstruction.

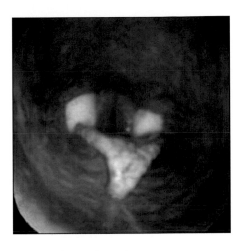

**Figure 8-14** White foam overflowing from the esophagus in a horse with esophageal obstruction.

- Usually, feed and fluid collect cranial to the obstruction. This is often seen during initial endoscopic examination, and masks the obstructed site (Figures 8-15, through 8-18).

✓ Fluid can be removed transendoscopically by suction.

✓ Collected feed should be removed before the nature of the obstruction is revealed.

✓ Solid collected feed should be removed by lavage (see treatment).

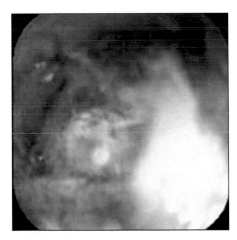 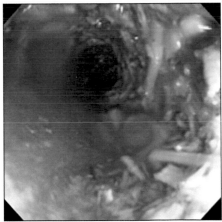

**Figures 8-15 and 8-16** Feed, bedding and fluid collected cranial to the esophageal obstruction, obscuring the site.

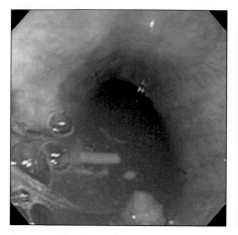
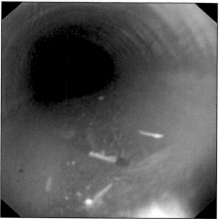

**Figures 8-17 and 8-18** Fluid collected cranial to the esophageal obstruction, obscuring the site of obstruction.

- If the obstruction is caused by feed (leafy alfalfa, coarse grass hay, grass, improperly soaked sugar beet), it is usually organized and appears as a bolus. (Figures 8-19 through 8-21).
- If the obstruction is caused by a sharp foreign body or has irregular edges (e.g. feeding bucket or wood fragments), an irregular shaped laceration may be seen around the feed that is collected cranial to the obstruction (Figures 8-22 and 8-23).
- Obstruction can also be caused by foreign bodies such as stones, bedding, medicinal boluses, carrots, apples, corncobs, potatoes (Figures 8-23 and 8-24).

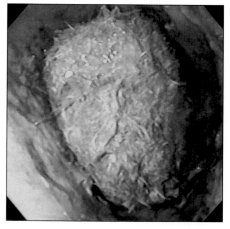
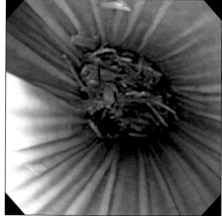

**Figure 8-19** Esophageal obstruction by feed at the post pharyngeal level.

**Figure 8-20** Esophageal obstruction by feed at the level of thoracic inlet.

**Figure 8-21** Esophageal obstruction by feed at the level of the base of the heart.

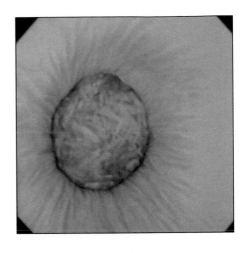

**Figure 8-22** Esophageal obstruction secondary to a sharp foreign body. Note the irregularly shaped laceration that is seen around the feed material that is collected cranial to the obstruction.

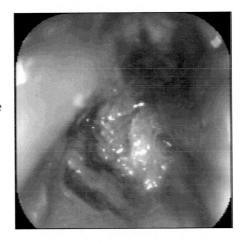

**Figure 8-23** A sharp foreign body was seen after esophageal lavage in the foal in figure 8-22.

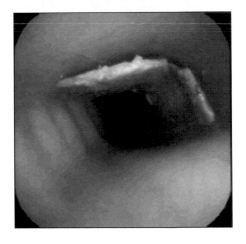

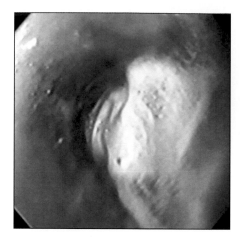

**Figure 8-24** Obstruction of the esophagus by a medicinal bolus in a foal.

🔖 In cases of failed or delayed gastric emptying, or gastric impaction, impacted feed may protrude through the cardia. This can look like an esophageal obstruction (choke). It is important not to mistake that appearance for esophageal obstruction (Figures 8-25 and 8-26).

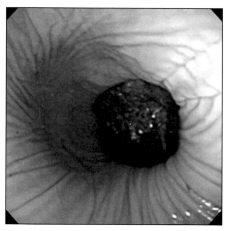

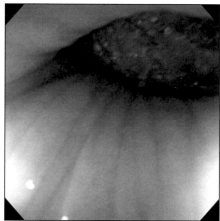

**Figure 8-25** Impacted feed protruding through the cardia in a horse that was suspected to have a delayed gastric emptying due to severe illness.

**Figure 8-26** Close up of figure 25.

# B-Secondary choke:

✓ Choke can occur secondary to other disease process.

✓ Secondary choke is caused by intraluminal or extraluminal abnormalities that mechanically impede feed passage.

✓ Intraluminal abnormalities include:

- **Esophageal stricture.**
- **Diverticulae.**
- **Cysts.**
- **Tumors.**

✓ Extraluminal obstruction by impinging on the esophagus:

- **Mediastinal and cervical masses (tumor or abscess).**
- **Vascular ring anomalies.**

✓ Endoscopic findings in secondary esophageal obstruction:

- Endoscopic examination of the esophagus first reveals feed and fluid collected cranial to the site of obstruction, which is similar to primary esophageal obstruction.

- In cases of extraluminal obstruction, the mucosa is intact but there is luminal stenosis, which is usually not circumferential.

- **Vascular ring anomalies** usually cause esophageal obstruction at the level of the heart base. It is a congenital condition, and foals show clinical signs when they start eating solid feed (Figures 8-27 and 8-28).

✓ **Esophageal stricture** appears as a circumferential narrowing of the esophageal lumen.

✓ A **diverticulum** appears as a focal out pouching of the intact mucosa:

- Two types: traction and pulsion diverticulum.
- Horses usually have recurrent choke episodes.

✓ In a traction diverticulum, the neck of the sac is much wider than the bottom. The sac can be viewed endoscopically (Figure 8-28).

- In a pulsion diverticulum, the neck of the sac is narrower than the bottom. It is usually impacted with feed and unless lavaged, cannot be visualized (Figure 8-29).

✓ Esophageal tumors are viewed as irregular or nodular masses in the lumen of the esophagus (eg. squamous cell carcinoma).

- The mucosa may appear ulcerated.

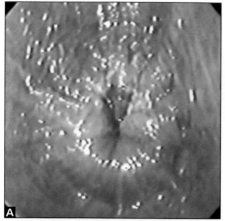

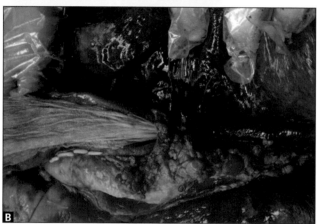

**Figure 8-27A,B** Vascular ring anomaly in a foal. A: Endoscopic appearance of the esophagus. B: Post mortem photograph. (Figure 8-27B, courtesy of Dr. M. Martinez).

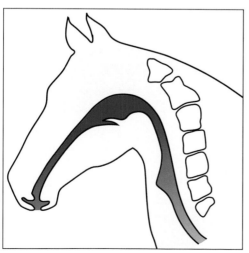

**Figure 8-28** Traction diverticulum.

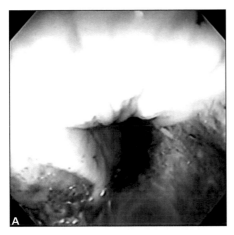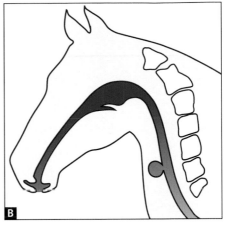

**Figure 8-29A,B** Pulsion diverticulum. A: Endoscopic appearance of an esophagus with a pulsion diverticulum. Note the feed that is impacted and filling the diverticulum while the esophagus is patent. B: A drawing of a pulsion diverticulum. (Photograph A, Courtesy Dr. A. Ruksznis).

♥ Esophageal cysts are usually seen as a protrusion from the mucosa of the esophagus, which appears intact but has transverse rather than longitudinal folds. This is usually where the cyst is located.

## Follow up

♥ Following resolution of the choke, endoscopic examination of the esophagus is important to determine whether ulceration, perforation, masses, strictures, or diverticulae are present. Endoscopic examination is also prognostically useful (Figures 8-30 through 8-34).

✓ Circumferential esophageal ulceration and ongoing esophageal inflammation is likely to form an esophageal stricture (Figure 8-35).

✓ When stricture is formed, feed modification should include only soft feed.

✓ Horses with esophageal stricture are more prone to recurrent esophageal obstruction.

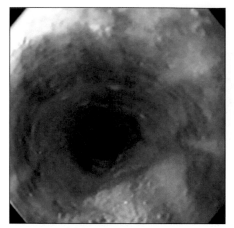

**Figure 8-30** Diffuse superficial ulceration of the esophagus in a foal after the obstruction was relieved. This type of ulceration is less likely to cause a stricture.

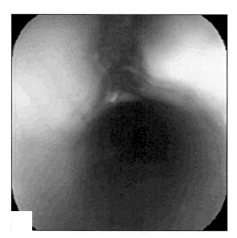

**Figure 8-31** Partial-thickness tear of the esophagus which was seen after relief of an obstruction in a foal. The foal recovered uneventfully.

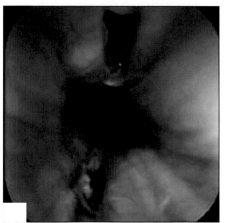

**Figure 8-32** Full thickness tear of the esophagus which was seen after the obstruction was relieved in a foal with an esophageal foreign body.

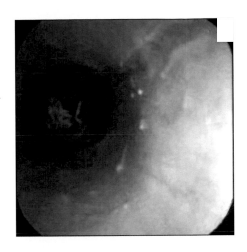

**Figure 8-33** Superficial, linear, ulceration of the esophagus. The horse recovered uneventfully. This kind of ulceration is less likely to cause an esophageal stricture.

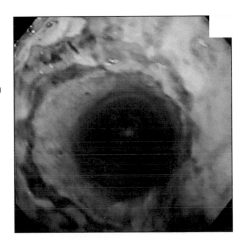

**Figure 8-34** Circumferential ulceration of the esophagus which was seen after relief of an obstruction in a horse. The horse had recurrent episodes of choke. It died after developing an aspiration pneumonia. This kind of ulceration is very likely to cause stricture of the esophagus.

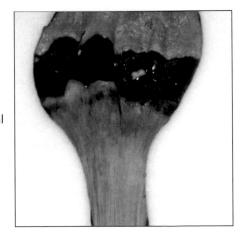

**Figure 8-35** A postmortem photograph of an esophageal stricture formed subsequent to a circumferential esophageal ulceration (Same horse as Figure 8-34).

# Treatment and Management

♥ Esophageal obstruction is an emergency situation and should be dealt with as soon as possible.

Most cases of primary esophageal obstruction resolve either spontaneously or with medical management.

✔ Unless the nature of the obstruction is known, there is no difference in the initial treatment and management between primary and secondary esophageal obstruction.

On presentation, the main treatment goals are:

• Sedation to reduce anxiety.

• Esophageal muscle relaxation to reduce esophageal spasm and allow passage of the impacted materials.

✔ Analgesics to reduce pain and anti-inflammatory agents to reduce inflammation of the esophagus.

☙ Correction of dehydration and acid base imbalances (especially important in chronic cases).

☙ Prevention or early detection and treatment of aspiration pneumonia.

☙ If the previous steps are unsuccessful, warm water can be pumped gently (using a stomach pump through a cuffed or uncuffed tube) into the esophagus cranial to the obstruction. The tube should be gently manipulated against the obstruction.

Manipulation of the tube should be done gently since rough handling may damage the esophagus.

Repeated attempts to relieve esophageal obstruction by lavage using a nasogastric tube, may cause nasal or pharyngeal bleeding. Blood may be swallowed and collect cranial to the obstruction (Figure 8-36).

✔ Water and impacted material often comes out of the nose or mouth of the horse during lavage and should be examined to determine the nature of the obstructing materials.

♥ Esophageal lavage can be performed in an anesthetized horse with an endotracheal tube in place with the cuff inflated (Figures 8-37 through 8-39).

♥ Esophageal lavage can also be performed in a standing horse, under profound sedation. Sedation is required to keep the head low and to prevent aspiration of fluids.

♥ Surgical removal and esophagotomy have many potential complications and should be considered as the last resort.

**Figure 8-36** Bloody fluid is seen in the esophagus cranial to an obstruction. The horse was swallowing blood from nasal bleeding during attempts to relieve the obstruction by lavage using a nasogastric tube.

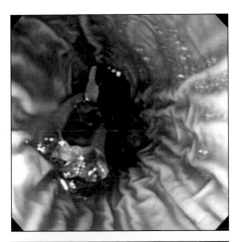

**Figure 8-37** An endotracheal tube is placed in the trachea with the cuff inflated to secure the airways and prevent aspiration. Another tube is passed into the esophagus to perform the lavage. This is a safe method of relieving an esophageal obstruction.

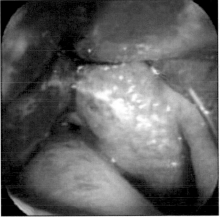

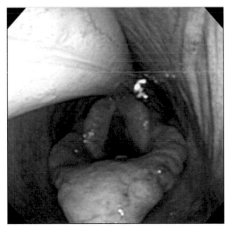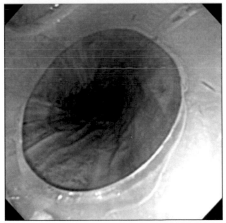

**Figures 8-38 and 8-39** An endotracheal tube is placed in the esophagus with the cuff inflated. A smaller diameter tube is passed through the endotracheal tube to perform the lavage.

✓ Endoscopy can also be used to retrieve foreign bodies (Figures 8-40 and 8-41).

♥ Complications of choke include esophageal ulceration, stricture, perforation, aspiration pneumonia, megaesophagus, and reobstruction (Figure 8-42).

♥ Esophageal endoscopy and ultrasonography should be performed after obstruction has been resolved to look for possible complications.

⌖ If esophageal ulceration or dilatation is found, the esophagus should be re evaluated every 2-4 weeks.

✓ Recurrence or reobstruction occurs in as high as 37% of cases.

✓ Reobstruction is usually predisposed by esophageal dilatation, mucosal injury, or esophagitis secondary to the initial esophageal obstruction.

✓ Depending on the duration of the obstruction and degree of damage, the recurrence rate is highest in the first 24-48 h. Feed should be withheld for the first 24 to 48 h post obstruction. After that, soft feed (moistened pellets and bran mashes) can be fed for about 7 days.

✓ In secondary esophageal obstruction, after removal of the collected feed and fluid cranial to the obstruction, treatment and management depend on the primary condition.

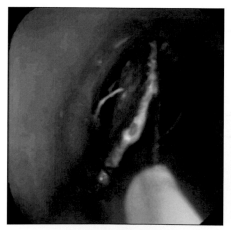

**Figure 8-40** An esophageal foreign body being retrieved using a snare.

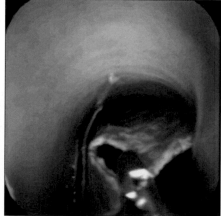

**Figure 8-41** Esophageal foreign body being retrieved using a forceps.

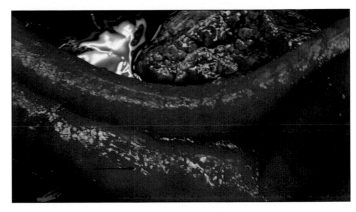

**Figure 8-42** Megaesophagus in a foal secondary to long standing esophageal obstruction. Arrow: esophagus.

# Esophagitis

✓ Esophagitis is seen as pink to red discoloration of the mucosa which can be intact or ulcerated.

✓ The lesion distribution depends on the cause. It can be focal, diffuse, or patchy.

✓ Reflux esophagitis causes lesions in the distal part of the esophagus and close to the lower esophageal sphincter.

Systemic conditions (eg. nonsteroidal antiinflammatory drugs toxicity) cause lesions throughout the esophagus. The lesion distribution appears organized (Figure 8-43).

✓ Esophagitis caused by *Candida albicans* can cause white or green tinged mucosal plaques.

**Figure 8-43** Circular mucosal lesions in the esophagus of a horse with phenylbutazone toxicity.

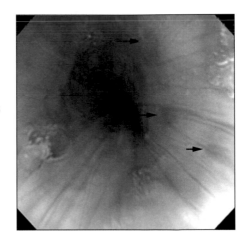

# Megaesophagus

✓ Usually secondary to long standing esophageal obstructions (Figure 8-42).

Endoscopic examination of the esophagus reveals an enlarged lumen that contains fluid.

✓ Peristaltic movements are reduced or absent.

✓ Insufflation of the esophagus leads to elongation, distortion, or misshaping of the lumen (Figure 8-44).

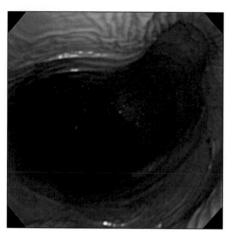

**Figure 8-44** Misshapen esophageal lumen after insufflation in a horse with megaesophagus. Note the collection of fluid in the lumen.

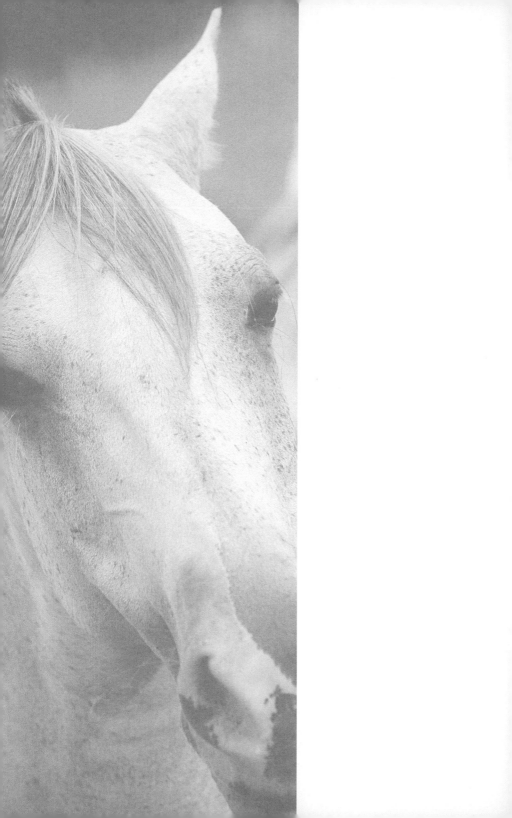

# Section 9
# Endoscopy of the Stomach

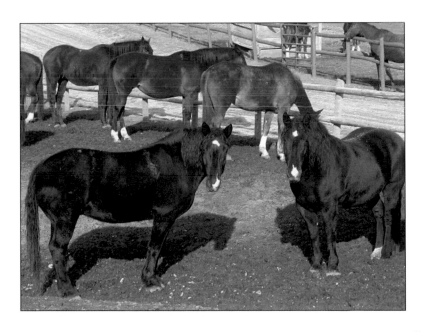

# Anatomy

The stomach has a capacity of 5 to15 liters.

Viewed from outside, the stomach looks like a bent pear and is divided into 4 parts; the cardia (entrance), fundus, body and pylorus (termination).

Viewed from inside, the stomach has different regions; the cardia, nonglandular region, margo plicatus, glandular region, and pylorus (Figures 9-1 and 9-2).

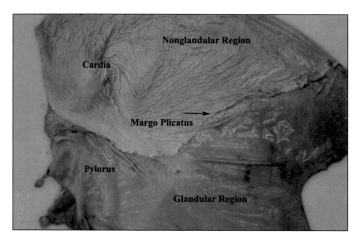

**Figure 9-1** An inside view of the anatomy of the stomach.

Food passage through the stomach is controlled by two sphincters; the cardia and pylorus.

The cardia and pylorus are quite close together.

✓ The short concave side between the cardia and pylorus is known as the lesser curvature, while the convex side between them is called the greater curvature.

✓ From the inside, a stepped edge (margo plicatus) divides the stomach into two parts; the non glandular and glandular region.

✓ The nonglandular region is slightly rough, white in color and occupies the fundus and part of the body of the stomach.

✓ The glandular part is smooth, reddish pink in color, and occupies the pylorus and the rest of the body of the stomach.

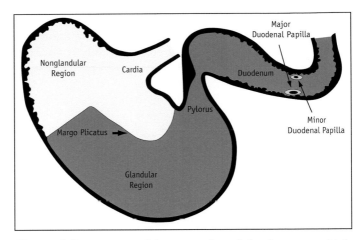

**Figure 9-2** Anatomy of the stomach and duodenum; sagittal section.

# Endoscopic Technique

♥ Feed should be withheld for 12 to 48 hours and water for 6 to 12 hours before examination.

✓ The animal should be properly restrained and sedated.

✓ The required length of endoscope depends on the size of the horse.

✓ In the adult horse, a 3 meter endoscope is recommended.

The endoscope is advanced to the end of the esophagus and passed through the lower esophageal sphincter into the stomach (Figure 9-3).

✓ Examination of the stomach should be done in a systematic way.

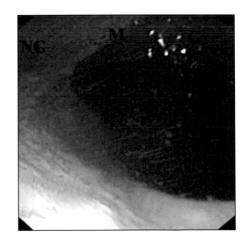

**Figure 9-3** Endoscopic view of the entrance of the stomach. NG – Nonglandular region, G – Glandular region, M – Margo plicatus.

After entering the stomach, the tip of the endoscope should be directed upward to view the nonglandular region and downward to view the glandular region of the stomach (Figures 9-4 through 9-7).

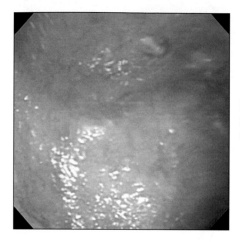

**Figure 9-4** Endoscopic view of the nonglandular region of a normal stomach.

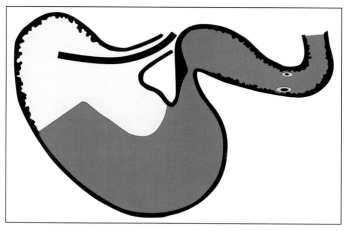

**Figure 9-5** The path and direction of the endoscope that corresponds to the view in Figure 9-4.

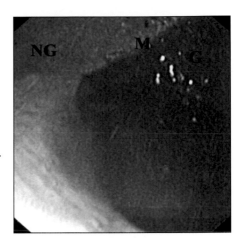

**Figure 9-6** Endoscopic view of the stomach. The tip of the endoscope is directed downward to view the glandular region. NG-Nonglandular region, G-Glandular region, M- Margo plicatus.

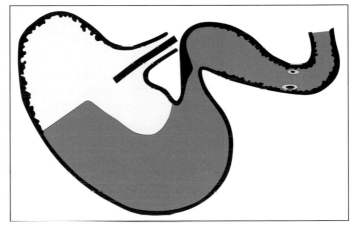

**Figure 9-7** The path and direction of the endoscope that corresponds to the view in Figure 9-6.

The fundus is readily seen when the stomach is entered (Figures 9-8 through 9-10).

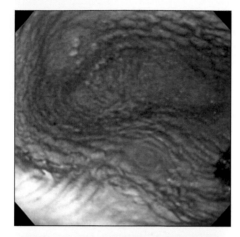

**Figure 9-8** Endoscopic view of the fundus of the stomach. The stomach is not fully inflated with air.

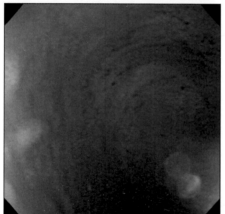

**Figure 9-9** Endoscopic view of the fundus of the stomach. Stomach is inflated with air.

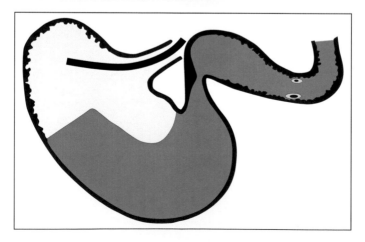

**Figure 9-10** The path and direction of the endoscope that corresponds to the view in Figures 9-8 and 9-9.

If the mucosa of the stomach is covered with residual feed material adhered to it, a 60 ml syringe can be attached to the biopsy channel and used to push water through to rinse the mucosa (Figure 9-11).

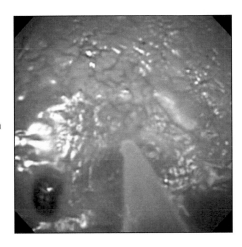

**Figure 9-11** Rinsing the mucosa of the stomach by pushing water through the biopsy channel.

♥ The stomach may be inflated by passing air through the air flush channel of the endoscope for better viewing.

The endoscope should be retroflexed in order to examine the cardia and the lesser curvature. This can be achieved by advancing the endoscope towards the center of the fundus while the tip is turned to the right. Turning the tip should be followed by continuous advancement of the endoscope until the cardia and the lesser curvature are seen. (Figures 9-12 and 9-13).

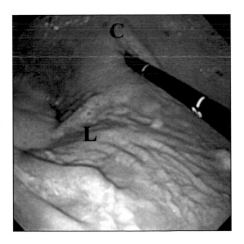

**Figure 9-12** Endoscopic view of the cardia and lesser curvature of the stomach. C – Cardia, L – lesser curvature.

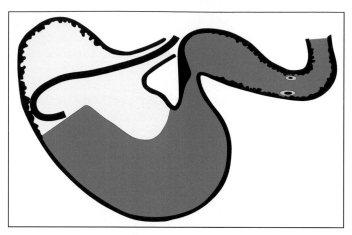

**Figure 9-13** The path and direction of the endoscope used to view the cardia and lesser curvature. This corresponds to the endoscopic view in Figure 9-12.

♥ To view the pyloric antrum and pylorus, the endoscope is advanced towards the margo plicatus and the tip should be turned downward just before it reaches the greater curvature. The endoscope is then advanced along the greater curvature until the pyloric antrum is seen (Figures 9-14 through 9-18).

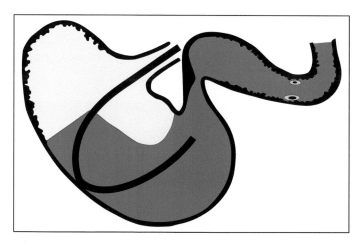

**Figure 9-14** The path and direction of the endoscope in order to view the pyloric antrum. This corresponds to the endoscopic view in Figures 9-15 through 9-18.

**Figure 9-15** Endoscopic view of the pyloric antrum of the stomach.

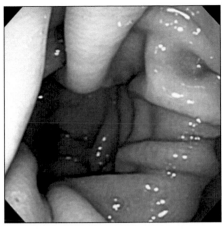

**Figure 9-16** Endoscopic view of the pyloric antrum of the stomach. Close up view of the pyloric opening (P).

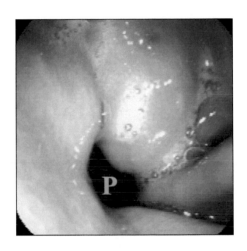

**Figure 9-17** Endoscopic view of the pyloric antrum of the stomach while contracting.

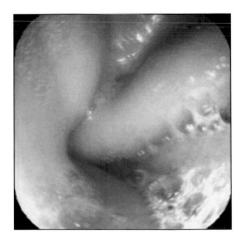

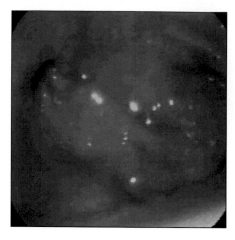

**Figure 9-18** Endoscopic view of the pyloric antrum of the stomach. The stomach is inflated with air.

✓ The presence of food and water may obscure the view of the pyloric antrum.

✓ If fluid is present and obscuring the view, it may be suctioned using a pump or a 60 ml syringe attached to the biopsy channel.

As in the nonglandular part of the stomach, if the mucosa is covered with residual feed material that is adhered to it, a 60 ml syringe can be attached to the biopsy channel and used to rinse the mucosa with water (Figure 9-19).

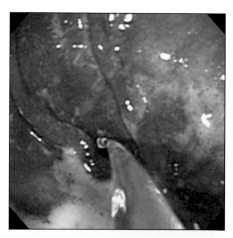

**Figure 9-19** Rinsing the mucosa of the stomach by pushing water through the biopsy channel.

# Normal Endoscopic Findings

Normal anatomical findings:

- The nonglandular region (Figures 9-4, 9-8, 9-9 and 9-14).
- The fundus (Figures 9-8 and 9-9).
- The cardia (Figure 9-12).
- The lesser curvature (Figure 9-12).
- The margo plicatus (Figure 9-6).
- The glandular region (Figures 9-15 through 9-19).
- The pyloric antrum and pylorus (Figures 9-15 through 9-18).

# Diseases of the Stomach

## Gastric Ulcers

✓ It is a multifactorial disease and the cause differs from case to case.

✓ It is mainly recognized in performance horses and sick foals.

✓ The disease does not seem to be associated with clinical signs in most affected animals.

✓ Endoscopically, it is usually described by location and severity.

Location:

- Glandular vs. nonglandular (squamous) region of the stomach (Figures 9-20 through 9-23).

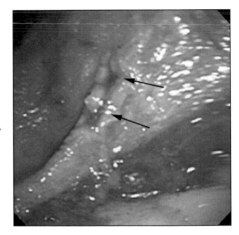

**Figure 9-20** Ulceration of the nonglandular region of the stomach (arrows).

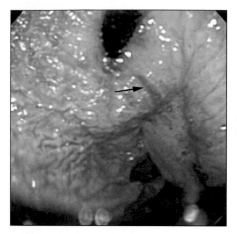

**Figure 9-21** Linear ulceration of the cardia, nonglandular region, of the stomach (arrow).

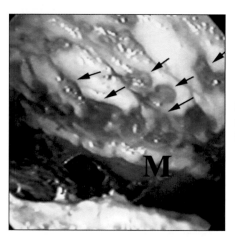

**Figure 9-22** Multiple ulceration of the nonglandular region of the stomach (arrows). M – margo plicatus.

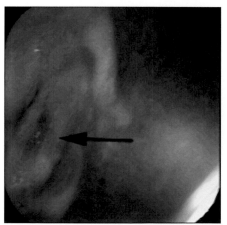

**Figure 9-23** Ulceration of the glandular region of the stomach (arrow). Courtesy of the Atlantic Veterinary College.

Severity (listed in increasing order).

✓ Desquamation of the squamous epithelium occurs in young foals and appears as flakes or sheets of epithelium.

✓ Erosion is a superficial lesion involving the mucosa only.

✓ Ulceration is a deeper lesion. It extends to the submucosal and deeper layers of the stomach.

# Endoscopic Findings and Appearance of Gastric Ulceration

✓ Desquamation of the squamous epithelium appears as flakes or sheets of epithelium.

☞ Ulcers and erosions are associated with loss of the mucosal epithelium causing a concave appearance of the stomach surface where the ulceration occurred. The lesion is surrounded by high margins.

☞ Erosions and ulceration may be linear, circular, irregular, or crater-like in shape (Figures 9-21, 9-24, and 9-29). Ulcers may coalesce (Figure 9-25).

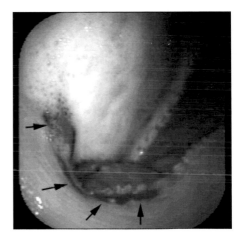

**Figure 9-24** Linear ulceration of the nonglandular region of the stomach (arrows).

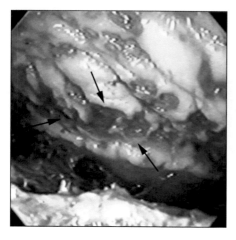

**Figure 9-25** Different shaped ulcerations of the nonglandular part of the stomach. Arrows point at a coalescent ulcer.

✓ The base of the ulcer or erosion is usually red in color, and can sometimes be seen as yellow, golden colored crusts.

✓ Glandular surface lesions may vary in appearance from a discrete defect in the mucosal surface to an area of roughening and hyperemia.

♥ Glandular surface ulceration may only be identified by the presence of an acute hemorrhage or brown material (denatured blood).

✓ Red and brown areas are seen when recent hemorrhage occurs.

✓ Thick white margins of an ulcer are an indication of healing (Figure 9-26).

Gastric ulceration has been scored based on the endoscopic appearance (Table 9-1).

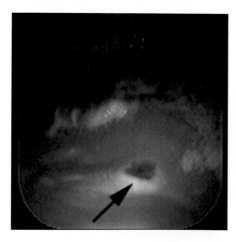

**Figure 9-26** Healing ulcer in the nonglandular region of the stomach (arrow).

Table 9-1

Practitioner's Simplified Scoring System
(Andrews *et al.* (1999), Equine Vet. J. Suppl., 29, 81-86)

| SCORE | LESION DESCRIPTION |
|-------|--------------------|
| 0 | Intact mucosal epithelium. It may have reddening and / or mild hyperkeratosis |
| 1 | Small single or small multifocal lesions |
| 2 | Large single or large multifocal lesions or extensive superficial lesions |
| 3 | Extensive, often coalescing lesions, with areas of deep ulceration |

# Clinical Syndromes

## Foals

✓ Clinical signs include bruxism, dorsal recumbency, salivation, interrupted nursing, diarrhea, and colic.

Clinical signs are observed in a minority of foals with lesions seen endoscopically.

✓ Ulceration can affect both, the glandular and non-glandular areas of the stomach. However, it is more common in the nonglandular area along the margo plicatus and lesser curvature.

✓ Glandular ulceration is the most clinically significant type of ulceration in foals.

✓ Most ulcerations of the glandular area are seen in the pyloric area or the body of the stomach.

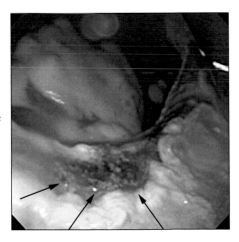

**Figure 9-27** Ulceration of the lesser curvature in the nonglandular region of the stomach (arrows).

# Yearlings and Adults

✓ Many horses with gastric ulcers, seen endoscopically, are clinically normal.

✓ Clinical signs vary and include anorexia and chronic or intercurrent abdominal discomfort.

✓ Other vague clinical signs that may be seen include decreased consumption of concentrates, postprandial episodes of colic, poor performance, or poor-quality hair coat.

Ulcers are most commonly seen in the nonglandular region of the stomach, but can also be seen in the glandular region (Figures 9-28 through 9-32).

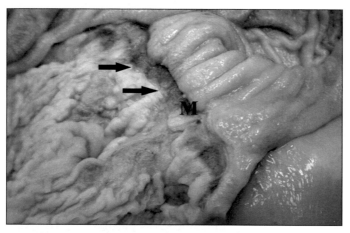

**Figure 9-28** Ulceration of the stomach (arrows) along the margo plicatus (M).

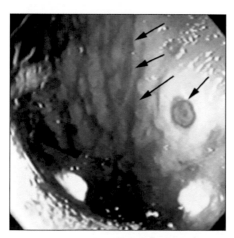

**Figure 9-29** Ulceration of the nonglandular region of the stomach (arrows).

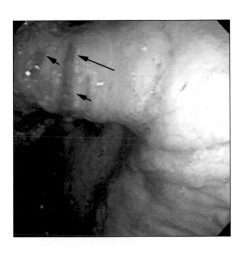

**Figure 9-30** Ulceration of the nonglandular region of the stomach (arrows).

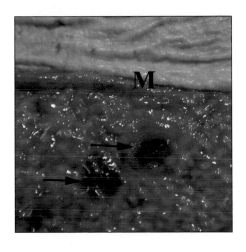

**Figure 9-31** Ulceration of the glandular region of the stomach (arrows). M – Margo Plicatus

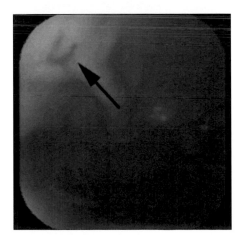

**Figure 9-32** Ulceration of the glandular region of the stomach (arrow). Courtesy of the Atlantic Veterinary College.

# Gastric Parasites

✓ Larvae of *Gasterophilus intestinalis*, "bots", may be seen in the stomach.

They are usually seen attached to the nonglandular surface, but may be attached to the glandular surfaces(Figures 9-33 through 9-35).

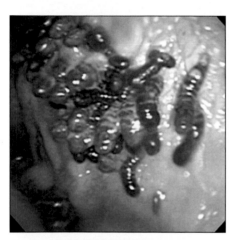

**Figure 9-33** Larvae of *Gasterophilus intestinalis*, "bots", attached to the nonglandular surface of the stomach.

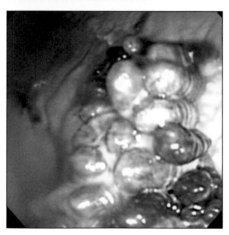

**Figure 9-34** Close up view of Figure 9-33.

They can be seen singly or in clusters most commonly adjacent to the margo plicatus (Figure 9-35).

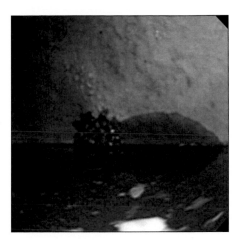

**Figure 9-35** A cluster of larvae of *Gasterophilus intestinalis*, "bots", attached to the glandular and nonglandular surface of the stomach adjacent to the margo plicatus.

✓ Larvae of *Gasterophilus nasalis* may be seen in the pylorus or proximal portion of the duodenum.

Lesions caused by *Draschia (Habronema) megastoma* may be seen as an intramural nodule of the gastric wall at the margo plicatus or on the glandular surface.

# Gastric Neoplasia

Gastric neoplasia is uncommon in horses.

✓ The most common gastric neoplasm is squamous cell carcinoma, which originates from the squamous epithelium (nonglandular region).

✓ Squamous cell carcinoma has a rough and nodular (cauliflower-like) appearance, with areas of ulceration and necrosis. There is usually a clear demarcation between normal and abnormal mucosa.

✓ Other reported neoplasms of the equine stomach include gastric adenocarcinoma, metastatic lymphosarcoma, mesothelioma, and bile duct carcinoma.

# Miscellaneous Gastric Conditions

✓ **Pyloric stenosis and secondary delayed gastric emptying** may be seen in the horse. It can be congenital due to hypertrophy of the pyloric musculature, or acquired secondary to abscessation, neoplasia, or duodenal ulceration and adhesions.

✓ **Impaired gastric emptying in foals** and secondary gastroesophageal reflux which can lead to the presence of a red or yellow color of the esophageal mucosa and esophageal ulceration.

**Gastric impaction** may be seen endoscopically by the presence of a bolus of compacted feed material protruding from the cardia (Figures 9-36 and 9-37).

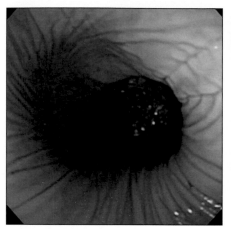

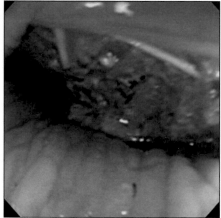

**Figure 9-36** A bolus of compacted feed material protruding from the cardia of the stomach. This can be seen in cases of gastric impaction or if the horse was not fasted prior to endoscopy.

**Figure 9-37** Close up view of Figure 9-36.

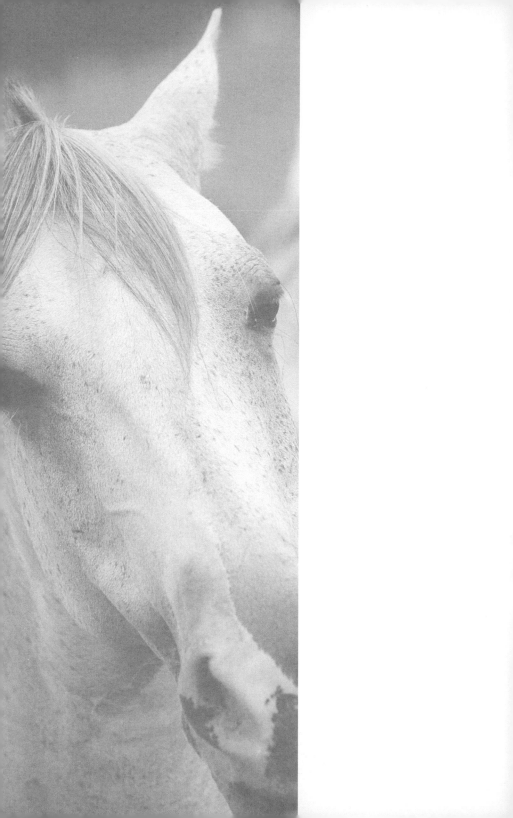

# Section 10

## Endoscopy of the Duodenum

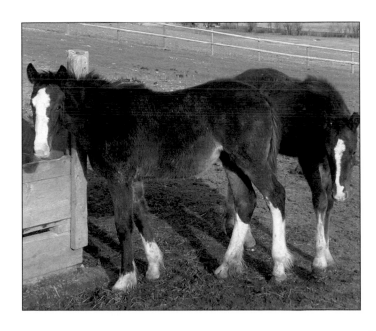

# Anatomy

The duodenum is a relatively short cylindrical structure (Figure 10-1).

It begins ventral to the liver where the cranial part forms a sigmoid flexure.

The first curve of the duodenal sigmoid flexure is convex dorsally and the second is convex ventrally.

✓ There are two duodenal papillae in the sigmoid flexure of the duodenum.

The major duodenal papilla, through which the bile and major pancreatic ducts discharge.

The minor duodenal papilla, through which the accessory pancreatic duct opens.

The major duodenal papilla is situated on the convex margin of the flexure, the minor duodenal papilla is on the facing margin (Figure 10-1).

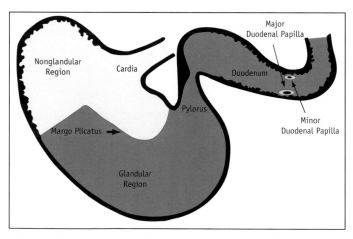

**Figure 10-1** Anatomy of the stomach and duodenum; sagittal section.

# Endoscopic Technique

✓ Preparation, restraint, and equipment required to perform duodenoscopy are similar to those used in gastroscopy.

✓ A three meter endoscope is required in the adult horse, while in weanlings, a 2.2 meter endoscope may be used.

✓ The same technique described for performing gastroscopy is used until the pylorus is visualized.

Once the pylorus is seen, the tip of the endoscope is directed toward the pyloric opening while advancing the endoscope (Figure 10-2).

✓ When the endoscope reaches the duodenal ampulla, advance slowly with the aid of gastrointestinal tract motility (peristalsis).

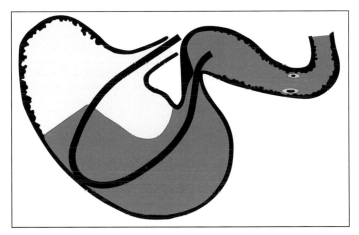

**Figure 10-2** The path and direction of the endoscope used to view the duodenum.

# Normal Endoscopic Findings

The duodenum is a cylindrical structure and very vascular.

The mucosa is reddish-brown in color with a velvety appearance and circular folds (Figure 10-3 and 10-4).

✓ The fluid in the duodenum is usually amber in color.

It contains the major and minor papillae. They are about 10-15 cm from the pylorus (Figure 10-5 through 10-9).

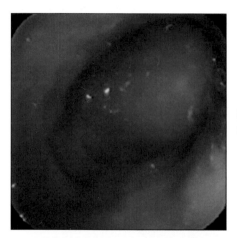

**Figure 10-3** Endoscopic view of the normal duodenum.

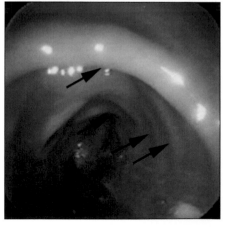

**Figure 10-4** Endoscopic view of the normal duodenum. Note the presence of the circular folds (arrows).

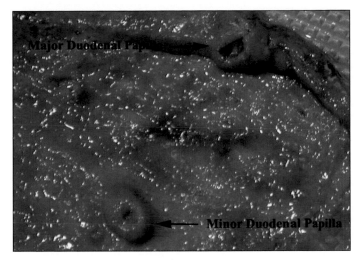

**Figure 10-5** The major and minor duodenal papillae in a post-mortem specimen.

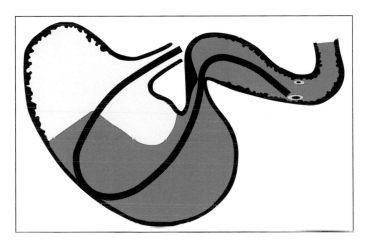

**Figure 10-6** The path and direction of the endoscope used to view the major duodenal papilla. This corresponds to the endoscopic view in Figure 10-7.

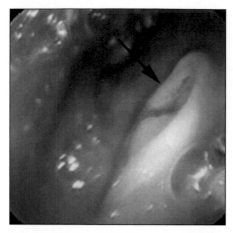

**Figure 10-7** Endoscopic view of the major duodenal papilla (arrow).

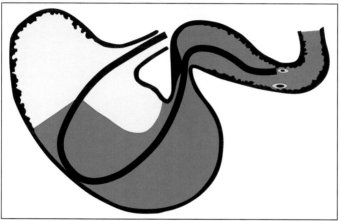

**Figure 10-8** The path and direction of the endoscope used to view the minor duodenal papilla. This corresponds to the endoscopic view in Figure 10-9.

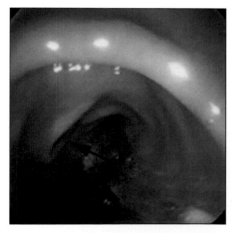

**Figure 10-9** Endoscopic view of the minor duodenal papilla (arrow).

# Diseases of the Duodenum

✓ **Duodenal ulcers** are usually associated with ulceration of the pyloric part of the stomach. This is usually referred to as gastro-duodenal ulcers.

✓ **Duodenal neoplasia, stenosis, diverticulae, and inflammation** have been reported.

✓ **Larvae of** *Gasterophilus nasalis* may be seen in the pylorus or proximal portion of the duodenum.

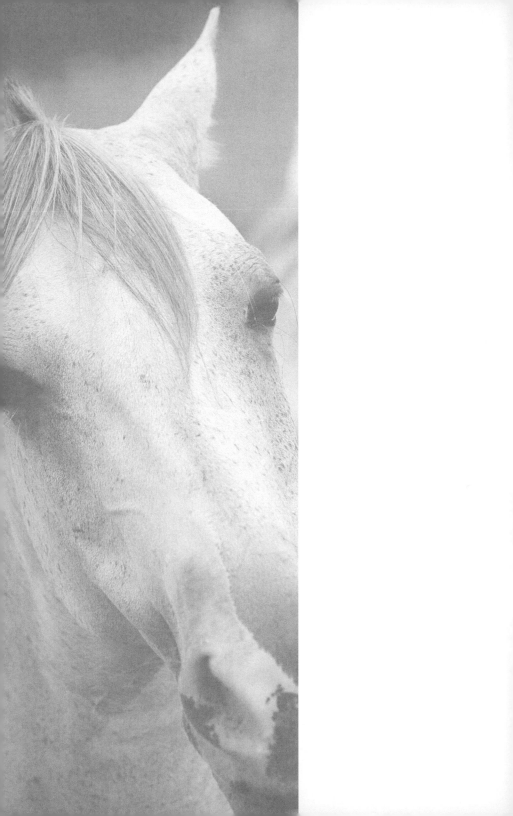

# Section 11

# Endoscopy of the Urethra, Bladder and Ureters

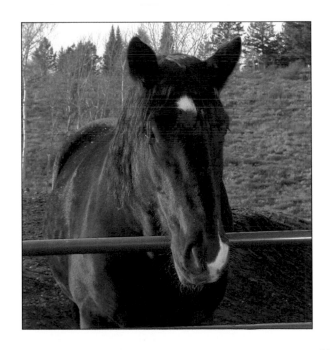

# Anatomy

The urinary system in the horse consists of two kidneys, associated ureters, a bladder and the urethra (Figure 11-1).

Each ureter is 6-8 mm in diameter.

The ureters connect with the bladder at the level of the bladder neck (trigone) (Figure 11-1).

✓ The bladder has a capacity of 3-4 liters of urine.

✓ In mares, the urethra is 2-3 cm long while in stallions and geldings, it is about 70-90 cm long.

✓ The colliculus seminalis and the openings of the prostatic ducts (two groups of papillae), lateral to the colliculus seminalis,

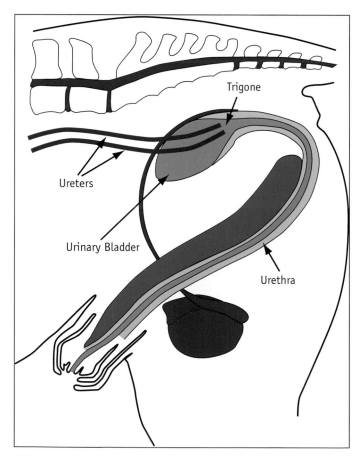

**Figure 11-1** Anatomy of the urinary tract in the horse.

are located immediately caudal to the urethral orifice, and dorsal in the pelvic urethra.

✓ The bulbourethral gland ducts are located a few centimeters caudal to the colliculus seminalis. The duct openings are seen as paired lines located dorsally.

✓ On the lateral aspect of the urethra, at the same level as the openings of bulbourethral gland ducts, the smaller openings of the lateral urethral gland ducts are located (Figures 11-4 and 12-4).

# Patient Preparation

The horse should be restrained and sedated to facilitate penile relaxation.

✓ Xylazine (0.04 mg/kg, IV) and acetylpromazine (0.02 mg/kg, IV) can be used to facilitate manual extension of the penis. The latter drug should not be used in stallions.

✓ The tail should be wrapped to prevent contamination during tail swishing.

✓ The sheath, penis, and urethral diverticulum should be cleaned in a routine fashion, using a warm solution of soft soap and water and cotton.

✓ In mares, the external genitalia should be cleaned and prepared in a similar fashion.

# Endoscopic Technique and Normal Endoscopic Findings

✓ The length of the endoscope should be ≥1 meter in length and ≤1 cm in diameter.

✓ The endoscope should be surgically scrubbed or chemically sterilized according to the endoscope manufacturer recommendation.

✓ To perform the endoscopy, two persons are required; an operator and assistant.

The tip of the endoscope (first few centimeters) should be aseptically lubricated.

The assistant should be wearing sterile gloves. The penis should be grasped proximal to the glans and keep it under gentle pressure.

In the mare, the urethral orifice should be identified digitally. The urethra is short and not readily examined. Urethral distension can not be achieved.

After grasping the glans penis in one hand, the assistant may introduce the aseptically lubricated endoscope into the penile urethra, with the other hand.

As directed by the operator, the assistant should pass the endoscope through the urethra.

♥ The assistant should maintain a pressure around the glans penis to occlude the urethra around the endoscope.

This will allow the distention of the urethra and bladder, and therefore a better visualization of the mucosa of the urinary tract.

✔ If the horse assumes the posture to urinate, the pressure around the glans penis should be reduced so the air and urine can come out. The penis should be directed down and the endoscope should be left in place (close biopsy portal).

✔ The endoscope should be advanced after emptying the bladder.

✔ The urethra is a tubular structure with pale pink mucosa that contains longitudinal folds. When distended the mucosa appears smooth and dark red in color (Figure 11-2A and B).

♥ Overdistension of the urethra will cause the blood vessels of the corpus spongiosum to be visible through the thinned urethral mucosa. The appearance may be mistaken for the presence of pathology (e.g. urethritis) (Figure 11-3).

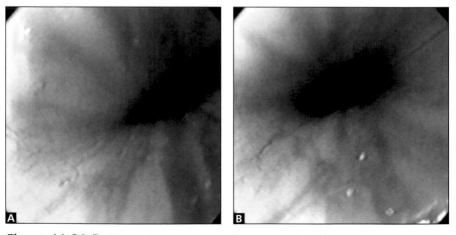

**Figure 11-2A,B** Mucosal appearance of the normal urethra.

**Figure 11-3** Mucosal appearance of the normal urethra when over-distended with air (arrows).

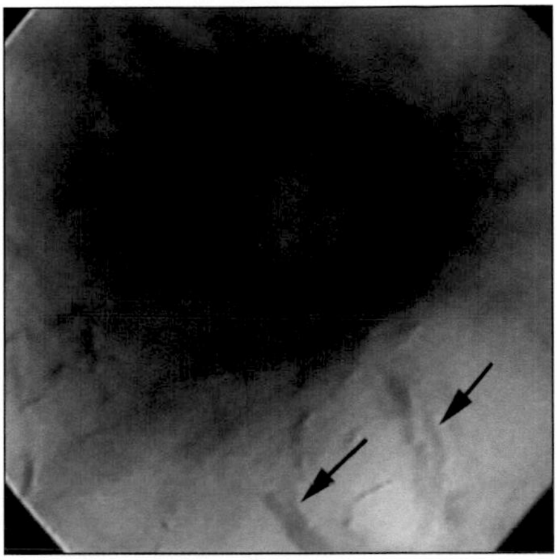

♥ In addition, overdistension of the urethra may interfere with identification of urethral lesions. If a lesion in the urethral mucosa is suspected, the air pressure should be released momentarily to visualize the suspected area of the urethra.

⌿ Repeated passage of the endoscope into the urethra may cause irritation and reddening of the urethral mucosa.

Once the endoscope reaches the ischiatic arch, it will enter the pelvic urethra.

♥ If the endoscope is rotated about 180°, the view will look inverted (up-side-down).

In the pelvic urethra the paired lines of the openings of the bulbourethral gland ducts are located dorsally and the smaller openings of the lateral urethral gland ducts are located lateral to the bulbourethral gland ducts but the same level (Figures 11-4, 12-4 and 12-8).

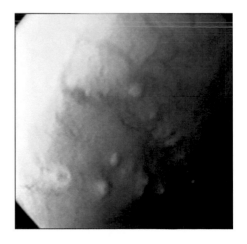

**Figure 11-4** The openings of the bulbourethral gland ducts.

♥ A few centimeters farther in the pelvic urethra, the colliculus seminalis and the openings of the prostatic ducts are located dorsally (in the roof of the urethra). The prostatic ducts are usually collapsed and not readily seen (Figures 11-5 and 12-5).

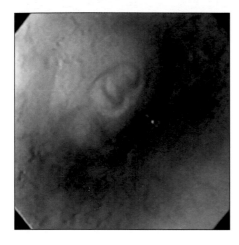

**Figure 11-5** The colliculus seminalis.

✔ The pelvic urethra terminates 2-3 cm proximal to the colliculus seminalis.

✔ Mild pressure might be needed to pass through the urethral sphincter.

✔ Once the bladder is reached orientation may be difficult.

✔ The urine pool should be present on the floor of the bladder, but if the endoscope was not rotated as described above, the urine pool will appear at the roof of the bladder (up-side-down) (Figures 11-6 and 11-7).

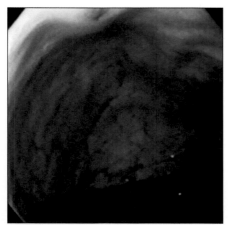

**Figure 11-6** Endoscopic appearance of the urine pool on the floor of the bladder.

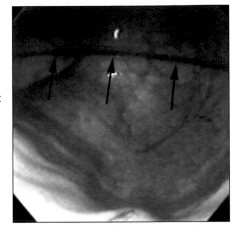

**Figure 11-7** Up-side-down endoscopic view of the urine pool that may be seen if the endoscope is not rotated (arrows).

✓ If the horse has not urinated and the bladder is full of urine (cloudy, dark yellow in color), visibility will be very poor. The bladder should be evacuated using suction through the endoscope (biopsy channel), or a separate catheterization may be done. Some clinicians catheterize the bladder prior to performing urinary tract endoscopy.

✓ The mucosa of the bladder is pale pink (redder than the urethra) (Figure 11-8).

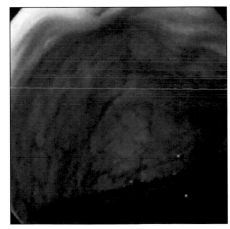

**Figure 11-8** Appearance of the normal mucosa of the bladder.

✔ A small diverticulum at the apex of the bladder is normal in some horses.

♥ The urinary bladder may be difficult to view if the endoscope is inserted too far or if the bladder is insufficiently distended.

✔ The tip of the endoscope should be withdrawn to the neck of the distended bladder to visualize the ureters.

Two slit-like uretral orifices can be seen in the dorsal part of the bladder (Figures 11-9 and 11-10).

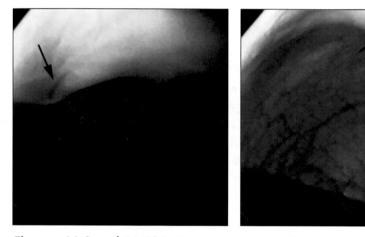

**Figures 11-9 and 11-10A** Normal appearance of the uretral opening (slit-like) (arrows).

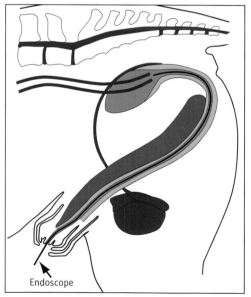

**Figure 11-10B** The path and direction of the endoscope corresponding to the view in Figures 11-9 and 11-10A.

After a few minutes, urine flow is observed exiting the ureteral orifices (Figures 11-11 through 11-13).

✓ If urine flow is not seen and the patients condition permits, diuretics may be administered to stimulate urine production.

✓ The ureters can be catheterized using the endoscope.

♥ The ureters of the mare are harder to observe because of the difficulty in maintaining the seal around the urethra so that the bladder can be fully distended.

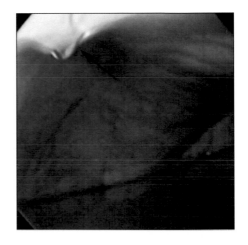

**Figure 11-11** Urine flow is observed exiting the left ureteral orifice (arrow).

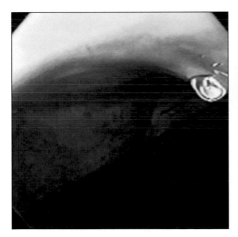
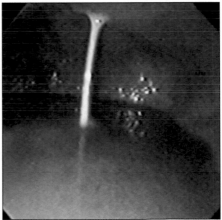

**Figures 11-12 and 11-13** Urine flow is observed exiting the right ureteral orifice (arrow).

# Diseases of the Urinary System

## Urolithiasis

✓ Urolithiasis is typically an adult horse disease and accounts for 7.8% of the diagnoses of urinary tract disease in the horse.

✓ Males, especially geldings appear to be predisposed to urolithiasis, and young race horses may be at higher risk because of NSAIDs use.

✓ The urinary bladder is the most common location for calculi (60%), followed by the urethra (24%), kidneys (12%), and ureters (4%).

✓ Incomplete obstruction is usually associated with dysuria, urinary incontinence, and mild abdominal pain.

Equine calculi are mainly composed of calcium carbonate and 90% of them are yellow-green in color, spiculated and easy to fragment. Ten percent are gray-white, smooth, difficult to fragment and contain phosphate in addition to calcium carbonate (Figures 11-14 and 11-15).

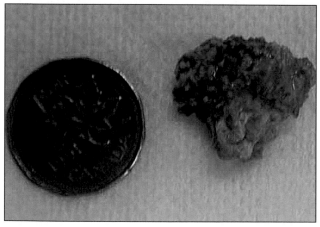

**Figure 11-14** A yellow-green, spiculated cystolith.

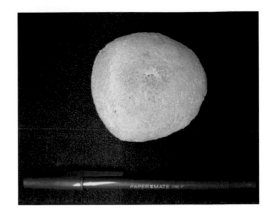

**Figure 11-15** A white, smooth cystolith.

# Cystolithiasis

♥ Hematuria following exercise is a common clinical sign. Other signs are pollakiuria, stranguria, urine incontinence or dysuria.

✓ Diagnosis is confirmed by transrectal examination, ultrasonography, and endoscopy.

Endoscopic appearance of the cystoliths (Figures 11-16 through 11-21).

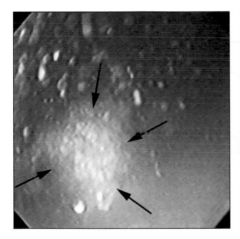

**Figure 11-16** Endoscopic appearance of a cystolith. The view of the cystolith (arrows) is not clear because the bladder is full of urine.

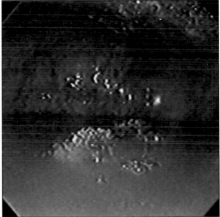

**Figure 11-17** Endoscopic appearance of a cystolith in the middle of a urine pool on the floor of the bladder.

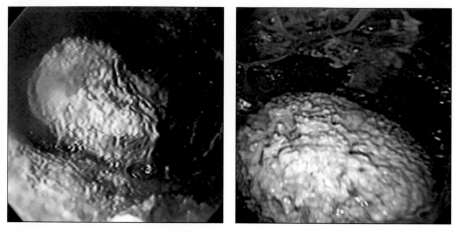

**Figures 11-18 and 11-19** Endoscopic appearance of a cystolith after the bladder is emptied. Note the cystitis that is associated with cystolithiasis in Figure 11-18.

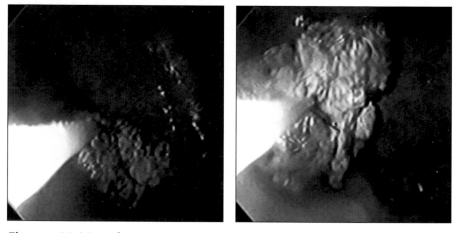

**Figures 11-20 and 11-21** Using a snare to remove a cystolith or break it down.

# Sabulous Urolithiasis

✓ Another form that has been described in the horse.

✓ It is characterized by accumulation of large amounts of crystalloid urine sediment (mainly calcium carbonate) in the ventral aspect of the bladder.

♥ It is usually caused by incomplete bladder emptying due to atony paralysis, caused by physical or neurological conditions.

♥ Affected horses usually present with urinary incontinence and ataxia of the hind limbs.

♥ Endoscopic examination of the bladder reveals large amounts of crystalloid urine sediment (white creamy to yellowish in color), that may appear as a mass, in the ventral aspect of the bladder (Figure 11-22).

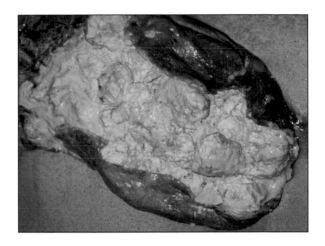

**Figure 11-22** Sabulous urolithiasis.

# Urethrolithiasis (Urethral calculus)

♥ Urethral calculus occurs primarily in male horses. It is usually caused by a small cystolith that passes from the bladder and lodges in the urethra, often in the area of natural narrowing of the urethra at the level of the ischial arch.

✓ Horses with urethral calculus present with signs of colic, frequent posturing to urinate, extension of the penis, dribbling small amount of urine, and sometimes blood at the end of the urethra.

♥ Unresolved complete obstruction can be followed by urinary bladder or urethral rupture.

✓ Diagnosis is based on clinical signs and the presence of a distended bladder and pulsating urethra on transrectal palpation.

Urethroscopy and careful palpation of the penis for a firm mass may also be diagnostic (Figures 11-23 through 11-26).

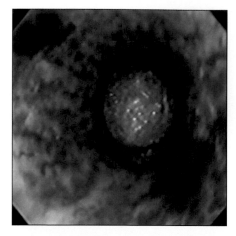

**Figure 11-23** Endoscopic view of a urethral calculus (urethrolithiasis).

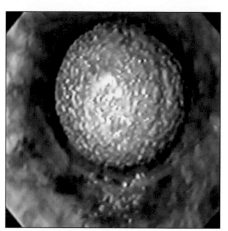

**Figure 11-24** Close up of Figure 11-23.

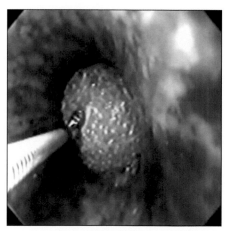

**Figure 11-25** Using forceps to evaluate the firmness and mobility of a urethral calculus.

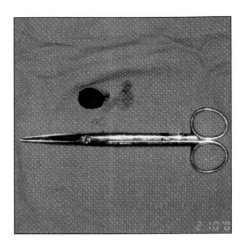

**Figure 11-26** Urethral calculus.

# Urinary Tract Infection

✓ Urinary tract infections are mainly ascending in origin (progress toward the kidney if untreated).

## Urethritis:

✓ Primary bacterial urethritis is undocumented in horses.

♥ The prominent vasculature and cavernosal spaces seen during urethroscopy may be mistaken for inflammation or even hemorrhage of the urethra (Figure 11-13).

✓ Traumatic, parasitic *(Habronemiasis)*, and neoplastic diseases of the urethra are known to occur (Figures 11-27 through 11-29).

✓ Repeated catheterization and cystolithiasis can result in urethritis.

*Habronema larvae* infestation can cause granuloma formation on the urethral process and consequent hematuria.

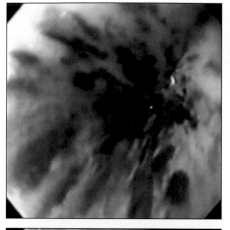

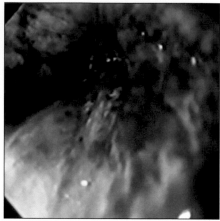

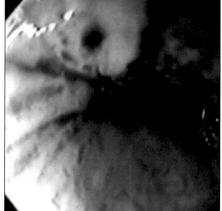

**Figures 11-27, 11-28 and 11-29**
Endoscopic view of the urethral mucosa in a horse with urethral calculus. Note the different degrees of urethritis and mucosal hemorrhages.

# Cystitis:

✓ Cystitis commonly occurs secondary to urinary flow disturbances caused by urolithiasis, bladder paralysis, neoplasia, anatomical defect, or iatrogenic trauma (catheterization or endoscopic examination).

✓ Clinical signs include hematuria, pollakiuria, stranguria, pyuria, or urine scalding of the perineum of mares or the front of the hind limbs of male horses.

✓ Diagnosis is based on physical examination, transrectal palpation, cystoscopy, ultrasonography, urinalysis and culture (Figures 11-30 through 11-34).

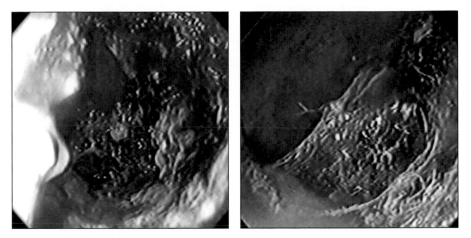

**Figures 11-30 and 11-31** Severe cystitis secondary to a bladder calculus in a mare.

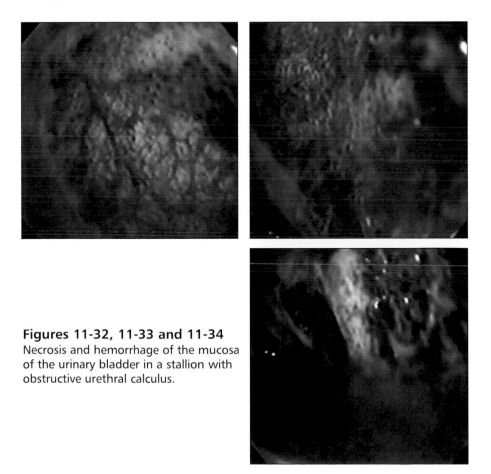

**Figures 11-32, 11-33 and 11-34**
Necrosis and hemorrhage of the mucosa of the urinary bladder in a stallion with obstructive urethral calculus.

## Pyelonephritis:

✓ Pyelonephritis has been associated with urolithiasis, cystitis, and bladder paralysis.

♥ Hematuria, pyuria (rather than stranguria and pollakiuria), weight loss, fever, anorexia, or depression are signs of

✓ Ureteral catheterization can be performed to assess if one or both kidneys are affected.

• It is not uncommon for pyelonephritis to be accompanied by ureteritis. The involved ureters are dilated and have poor smooth muscle tone (Figure 11-35).

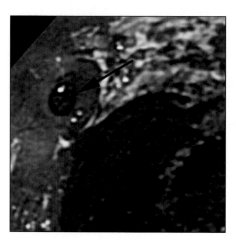

**Figure 11-35** Dilated ureteral opening, with poor smooth muscle tone in a case of ureteritis.

# Urethral Rent or Defect

This occurs on the dorsocaudal aspect or the convex surface of urethra at the level of the ischiatic arch (Figures 11-36 through 11-38).

Ureteral defects cause hematuria in geldings and hemospermia in stallions. Hematuria is typically at the end of urination.

✓ Quarter Horses or Quarter Horse crosses are most often affected.

✓ The exact cause is unknown. It has been suggested that contraction of the bulbospongiosus muscle during ejaculation or urination results in a "blowout" of the corpus spongiosum penis (vascular tissue surrounding the urethra) into the urethral lumen.

✓ Often, urethral rents heal without treatment. If hematuria persist more than a month, or the gelding become anemic, surgical treatment should be employed.

✔ Two surgical approaches are available for treatment of urethral rent; temporary ischial urethrotomy or making a vertical incision that extends into the corpus spongiosum penis but leaves the urethra intact.

♥ Urethrotomy may lead to stricture formation in the urethra. Hematuria should resolve within a week of surgical treatment.

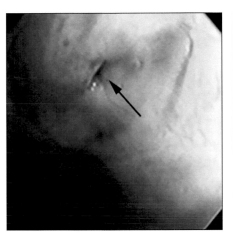 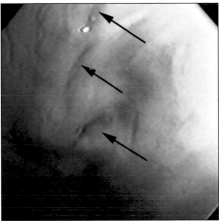

**Figure 11-36 and 11-37** Urethral defect(s) (arrows).

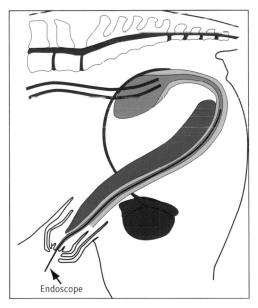

**Figure 11-38** The path and direction of the endoscope corresponding to the view in Figures 11-36 and 11-37.

# Idiopathic Renal Hematuria

💣☀ Idiopathic renal hematuria is associated with sudden onset, often life threatening, unilateral or bilateral renal hemorrhage.

No other signs of disease have been reported even with histological examination of affected kidneys.

✓ It is usually diagnosed after exclusion of other causes of hematuria. More than 50% of affected cases are Arabians.

✓ Diagnosis may also be made by using the endoscope to visualize blood exiting the ureter that corresponds to the affected kidney.

# Exercise-Associated Hematuria

✓ Commonly, hematuria associated with exercise is microscopic and not observed. In severe cases visible hematuria may occur. It is thought to be traumatic in origin, produced by the abdominal contents pounding the bladder against the pelvis during exercise.

✓ It is thought to be more common in horses that empty the bladder before exercise.

✓ Diagnosis is based on history of exercise and the presence of erosions or ulcers with a countercoup distribution on endoscopy.

# Urinary Tract Neoplasia

Urinary bladder tumors are uncommon conditions in the horse.

✓ Squamous cell carcinoma and to a lesser extent transitional cell carcinoma are the most common bladder tumors.

✓ Patients present for hematuria and / or stranguria. Palpable masses are felt on transrectal examination.

Endoscopic examination reveals tumor masses protruding from the wall of the bladder.

# Ectopic Ureter

✓ Ectopic ureter is rare in horses but much more frequently reported in females.

✓ It usually results in urinary incontinence since birth. Urine scalding of the hind limbs and the perineal area is common (in females).

In some cases, the only presenting complaint is urinary tract infection.

It can be unilateral or bilateral.

✔ The ureter may terminate in the vagina, cervix, or uterus (in mares) or beside the normal urethral orifice.

♥ In males, if the ureter terminates beside the normal urethral orifice urinary incontinence may not be seen because urine will enter the urethra and be controlled by the external urethral sphincter. The urine may also flow back to the bladder.

✔ Affected horses may be incontinent and have episodes of normal urination.

✔ Episodes of normal urination may be seen if a bladder fill occurs because of the urine carried by the normal ureter (unilateral ectopic ureter), or by retrograde flow from the urethra (ectopic ureter that terminates beside the normal urethral orifice).

✔ If the ectopic ureter terminates in the vagina, it may be visualized during endoscopy. The endoscope is passed into the vulva, while holding the labia closed so that the vestibule and vagina can be air-distended. This may allow visualization of intermittent urine flow exiting the ectopic ureter. The urine can be stained by systemic administration of fluorescein (11 mg/kg, IV), to better visualize the urine exiting the ectopic ureter.

# Urethrorectal Fistula

Urethrorectal fistula is a rare condition.

✔ It is usually seen in male foals but has been reported in an adult gelding.

It is thought to be congenital.

✔ It can be seen alone or with other congenital anomalies.

✔ Clinical signs include urine exiting through the anus.

A urethral defect or rent can be seen during endoscopy.

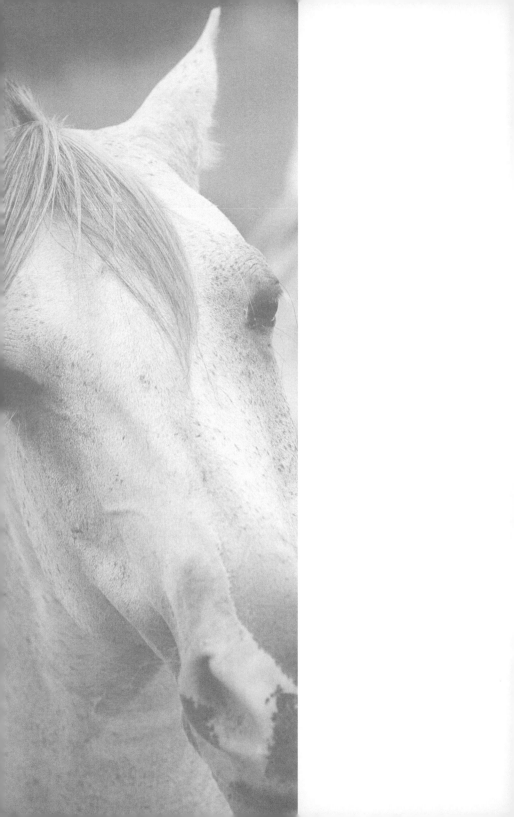

# Section 12

# Endoscopy of the Reproductive System of the Stallion

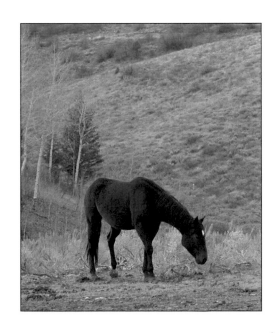

# Normal Anatomic Features

✓ The portions of the stallion's reproductive tract that may be assessed using endoscopy include the sheath, urethral opening (Figure 12-1), penile urethra, pelvic urethra, colliculus seminalis, and bladder. The Common Ducts of the ampullae and seminal vesicles open on the Colliculus Seminalis. Prostatic ducts, and Urethral glands, are visible along the urethra and the opening to the bladder is also visible.

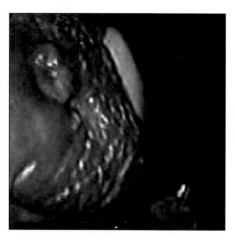

**Figure 12-1** Endoscopic view of the glans penis and urethral opening.

# Prepuce

✓ The penis of the stallion in the non-aroused state or gelding is retracted and located in the prepuce, which is also referred to as the sheath. The prepuce of the stallion is long and has a telescoping anatomic arrangement, or double invagination when retracted. The prepuce is divided into an external and internal portion. The external prepuce is adjacent to the scrotum. The opening to the prepuce on the ventral abdomen is called the preputial orifice. The internal prepuce has two portions called lamina. The internal lamina of the internal prepuce attaches to the shaft of the penis and at the preputial ring it joins the external lamina of the internal prepuce. The prepuce contains secretory tissue with glands that secrete smegma, a waxy substance.

✓ The external preputial cavity begins on the caudal ventral abdomen near the scrotum and extends to the preputial ring. The region from the preputial ring to the penis is the internal preputial cavity. The exterior and interior portion of the sheath of stallions and geldings may be visualized in situ using an endoscope for a short distance. The glans penis is immediately visible in the interior. For this reason the external lamina, internal lamina of the internal prepuce and glans penis are best examined by using sedation and mild traction to fully extend the penis and prepuce.

♥ If the goal is to fully assess the penis and internal and external preputial lamina, the stallion may be sexually aroused by teasing mares in estrus and/or sedated to allow the penis to drop. Geldings are usually sedated. Some tractable male horses allow the penis to be manually pulled down from the internal preputial cavity. Alpha agonists such as xylazine, and detomidine are useful for the purpose of sedation, and may be combined judiciously with acepromazine. Caution is advised when using acepromazine, because it has been reported to be associated with penile priapism.

♥ Sedation results in muscular relaxation, and allows the penis to protrude from the sheath. Indications for evaluating the interior of the sheath of a stallion/gelding include: history of never dropping the penis, excess discharge, foul smell, trauma, palpable mass, phimosis etc.

♥ Space occupying masses on the penis may prevent penile protrusion. In these cases endoscopy of the prepuce may be used. Conditions of the prepuce include: tumours such as squamous cell carcinoma, melanoma, lymphosarcoma, and sarcoids. Balanitis (infection or inflammation of the prepuce) may accompany coital exanthema, trauma or other bacterial infections.

☞ **Squamous cell carcinoma** is the most common tumour of the external genitalia in horses. Males are more commonly affected than females. There are usually multiple lesions located on the internal preputial lamina, penis and glans. Breeds of horses with little skin pigment such as appaloosas, and paint horses, or light coloured horses such as cremellos and buckskins are more commonly affected. Exposure to ultraviolet radiation from the sun is believed to be an inciting cause. Surgery, cryotherapy, chemotherapy (topical 5-Fluorouracil), and radiation therapy have been used to treat lesions.

♥ **Squamous papillomas** often accompany squamous carcinoma. The invasive nature of this tumour may result in extensive tissue destruction, and malodorous bloody preputial discharge. These tumours have a low grade of malignancy and surgical excision is frequently used to treat the condition. Topical treatment of squamous papilloma lesions with 5-Fluorouracil has been successful.

### Melanoma

⊶ Melanoma is an invariably malignant condition in horses. The tumours are common in the ventral tail, and perineal (perianal) tissue areas of grey horses. They are found in the parotid salivary gland. They are usually firm grey nodular dermal masses that are locally invasive, and over time metastasize. Surgical debulking or H2 receptor blockers have been reported to control the spread of the tumours.

### Lymphosarcoma

♥ Cutaneous lymphosarcoma may cause firm dermal masses in horses. Diagnosis is made by biopsy and or aspiration.

### Sarcoids

✓ Sarcoids are tumours that have 5 classifications: occult, verrucous, fibroblastic, nodular and mixed. They frequently occur on the head, limbs, and ventral abdomen of horses. They have been described on the prepuce of horses.

## Penis

The penis of a light horse stallion is approximately 50 cm long. The penis is approximately 6 cm in diameter. There is a large degree of variation in penile length and diameter.

### Penile Hypoplasia

✓ A history of never having seen the penis dropped has been reported due to penile hypoplasia that accompanied Persistent Mullerian Duct Syndrome in a horse. The horse had no history of castration and had the phenotypic appearance of a gelding. The shaft of the penis was very short which mechanically would not allow the penis to protrude from the sheath.

✓ Smegma and exfoliated skin debris is a normal finding in the sheaths of stallions. Loose skin debris accumulates at the preputial ring. Discharge from the sheath may be noted. Some discharge is attributed to normal preputial secretions, but excess secretion may accompany overzealous cleansing, bacterial overgrowth, balanitis, coital exanthema, foreign bodies, habronemiasis, and squamous cell carcinoma.

✓ Foreign bodies include stallion rings, misplaced rubber bands from malfunctioning artificial vaginas, and organic matter.

# Urethra

✔ The urethra in the stallion begins at the neck of the bladder, and ends on the ventral portion of the glans penis. Indications for evaluating the urethra include: hematuria, hemospermia, abnormal urination, pyspermia, fertility problems, and palpable accessory gland abnormalities.

☞ The urethra may be examined in its full length using a flexible gastroscope or videoendoscope that is 100 cm long (Figure 12-2). The urethra is surrounded anatomically by a vascular compartment called the corpus spongiosum. Sterile lubricant is applied to the sides but not the front of the endoscope. Sterile water or saline should be used to rinse the endoscope during viewing. The endoscope is advanced slowly through the urethra with low or intermittent airflow. The urethra should appear collapsed at the end of the field of view. This optimizes the chance of observing the urethral lesions. Once the lesion has been located more insufflation may be used to determine the extent of the injury. Over-dilation of the urethra is the most common error. The urethra will have a blanched appearance when over insufflated. Blood may be observed to rush back and forth in response to changing insufflation pressures. The blanching of the urethra may be confused with urethritis, and the movement of blood misidentified as hemorrhage (Figure 12-3). The degree of penile relaxation and length of the penis will determine the distance to the accessory sex gland openings and the bladder.

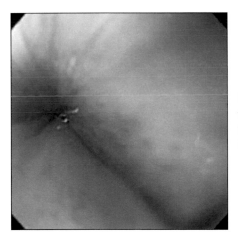

**Figure 12-2** View of the urethra with the recommended degree of insufflation. The mucosa should appear pink and the lumen should not be dilated.

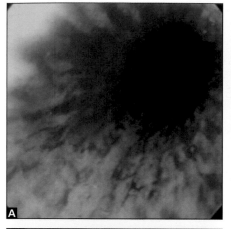

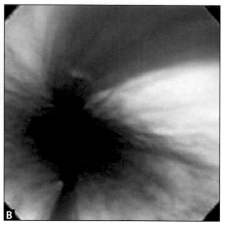

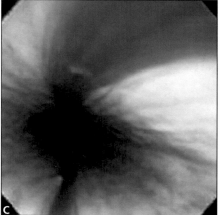

**Figure 12-3A-C** Panel A-C, Healthy but over-insufflated urethras. Panel A shows excessive urethral dilation and blanching of the mucosa, Panels B and C show artifactual pooling of blood in vessels that is easily confused with hemorrhage.

✓ Only after the full extent of the urethra has been examined is the insufflation pressure increased to allow viewing of the pelvic urethra and associated structures. As the endoscope is advanced over the brim of the pelvis, anatomic structures will come into view in sequence. The openings for the bulbourethral glands (Figure 12-4B) are found on the midline, followed by laterally located urethral glands (Figure 12-4A). Small openings of the prostatic ducts are visible near the colliculus seminalis (Figure 12-5). The common ducts of the ampullae and seminal vesicles can be seen opening on the colliculus seminalis. The distant slit-like structure is the opening to the bladder.

Variations in normal anatomy exist (Figures 12-7 and 12-8).

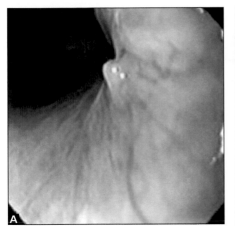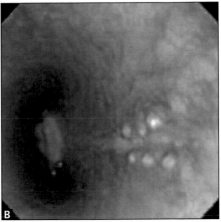

**Figure 12-4A,B** View of a dilated urethra as the junction between the pelvic and penile urethra. Panel A shows a laterally located urethral gland opening. Dorsal is to the right in Panel B. In Panel B the the bulbourethral glands' openings are large papilla like structures oriented in rows, the small urethral glands run laterally to these openings. Visible is the mound like colliculus seminalis with the openings of the 2 common ducts of the seminal vesicles and ampulla.

**Figure 12-5** View of the dilated pelvic urethra near the opening to the bladder showing the colliculus seminalis, common ducts, and bladder opening.

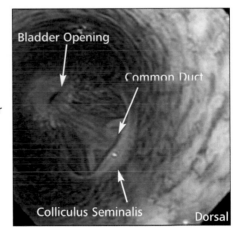

183

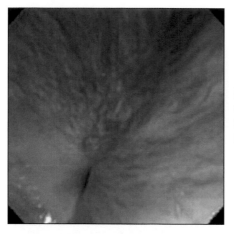

**Figure 12-6** A view of the opening to the bladder from the pelvic urethra. Note the change in colour of the mucosa at the neck of the bladder.

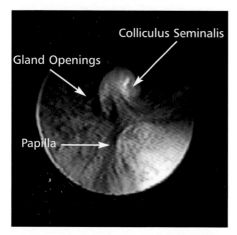

**Figure 12-7** Prominent papilla like gland opening (mound in the foreground), prominent colliculus seminalis, with additional gland openings craniad to the colliculus seminalis.

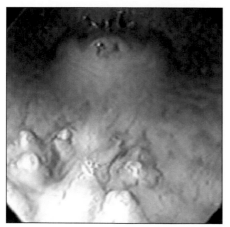

**Figure 12-8** Non-row like orientation of bulbourethral gland openings.

# Pathologic Conditions

## Urethritis

✓ Urethritis means inflammation of the urethra (Figure 12-9). The caudal segment of the urethra is usually involved. Accumulations of smegma forming small concretions (beans) in the urethral fossa may mechanically impinge on the urethral opening causing irritation. Bacterial infection of the caudal urethra may also be present.

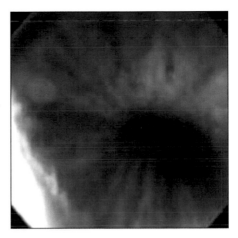

**Figure 12-9** Caudal urethritis - Image shows pinpoint hemmorrhages and tissue discolouration.

## Summer Sores–Habronemiasis of the Urethra

♥ **Habronemiasis** is cause by the hatched larva or Drashia spp and Habronema spp. The flies are attracted to moist tissue such as the prepuce and urethral opening. The lesions are pyogranulomatous and may be rapidly progressive. Scrapings of the affected tissue may contain larvae. Biopsies have characteristic features such as a dramatic eosinophilic infiltrate, and may be used to differentiate habronemiasis from squamous cell carcinoma. Caseous granules are present in the lesions. Complete blood counts may show systemic eosinophilia. Systemic and topical treatment with ivermectin, and non-steroidal antiinflammatory agents are used for treatment. Corticosteroids are used to decrease the immune response to the larvae.

# Seminal Vesiculitis

✔ This is an uncommon condition of stallions that is believed to be caused primarily by an ascending bacterial infection. One or both seminal vesicles may be affected. In cases of seminal vesiculitis, the seminal vesicles may or may not be enlarged on rectal examination, or have an abnormal echotexture (on ultrasound).

♥ A proportion of the mares bred to a stallion with seminal vesiculitis may develop a sexually transmitted bacterial endometritis caused by the same organism. Neutrophils may be identified in the semen. Mares may have short interestrous intervals. Semen should be sent for quantitative bacterial culture and sensitivity. The semen may show mixed bacterial growth. Pathogens associated with seminal vesiculitis include Klebsiella and Pseudomonas, however these organisms may be present in a commensal fashion. In the absence of clinical signs, recovery of these bacteria from the semen is not a significant finding. Palpation of the infected seminal vesicle during endoscopy may result in discharge coming from the common duct on the infected side (Figures 12-10 through 12-12). The common duct of the seminal vesicle is catheterized under endoscopic and rectal guidance to treat the tissue (Figure 12-14). The seminal vesicle is an organ where it is difficult to achieve good tissue concentrations of antibiotics (Figure 12-13). Local instillation of antibiotics has been reported to be beneficial. Semen extenders may be prepared with antibiotics that have activity against the bacterial contaminants. Discharge may or may not be seen coming from the common duct into the urethra.

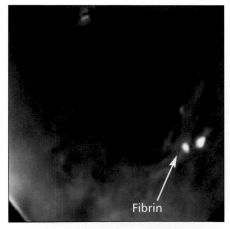

**Figure 12-10** Fibrin strand coming from the left common duct in a stallion with seminal vesiculitis.

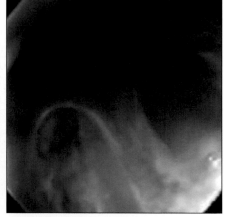

**Figure 12-11** Close-up view of brownish discharge coming from the common ducts.

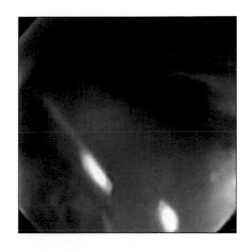

**Figure 12-12** View of purulent brown discharge coming from the right common duct of a stallion with seminal vesiculitis.

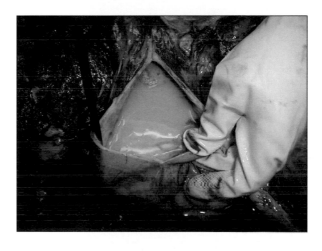

**Figure 12-13** Purulent discharge in a seminal vesicle at necropsy.

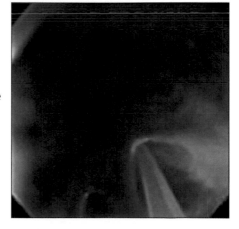

**Figure 12-14** A catheter is placed in the common duct and directed into the seminal vesicle. The catheter is used to flush the infected gland and to locally deliver antibiotics.

# Hemospermia

♥ Hemospermia - May be caused by trauma, idiopathic urethral rents, ulcers, and granulomatous lesions. Hemospermia may be micro or macroscopically visible. The chief complaint is usually frank blood on the stallion at dismount or on collection (Figure 12-15).

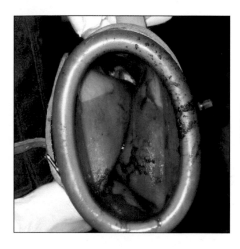

**Figure 12-15** Hemospermia: Blood in a Missouri style artificial vagina following semen collection.

Frank blood in the ejaculate causes infertility. The rule outs include problems that result in the mare's blood on the stallion including breeding injuries such as vaginal wall lacerations of the mare, and rupture of hymen. Blood may enter the ejaculate from the stallion from penile/preputial injuries, or urethral problems. There may be a history of trauma such as breeding through a fence or unsuccessfully jumping over a fence with a full erection. The most common cause of hemospermia is idiopathic hemospermia. The urethra is very vascular. During sexual arousal blood flow to the penis and urethra increases and pressure rises. A urethral lesion will communicate with the underlying corpus spongiosum penis and the pressure from sexual arousal will result in urethral bleeding. Sexual activity or arousal will prevent the lesion from healing. Bacterial infections of the urethra cause a distal primary urethritis, or an ulcerated area may be secondarily infected. Raised granulomatous lesions are sometimes seen.

⚷ For the purposes of diagnosis and prognosis of hemospermia a stallion should be sexually aroused to determine if blood drips from the penis. Semen collection should be performed if blood is not observed, as maximal penile and urethral pressures are achieved prior to ejaculation. Urethroscopy is used to determine the cause, location and extent of the urethral lesion. The most common location for urethral lesions associated with hemospermia is at the junction of the penile and pelvic portions of the urethra (Figures

12-16 through 12-20). This area is difficult to evaluate. It should be repeatedly and carefully evaluated with low urethral insufflation to initially identify the lesion. Over insufflation should be avoided, because the artefacts associated with over insufflation make the identification of urethral lesions very difficult. Once the location of the lesion has been identified moderate insufflation may be used to determine the depth and extent of the urethral lesion. Treatment includes: absolute sexual rest 3 weeks, with antibiotics added based on culture and sensitivity of the bacteria recovered from the lesion or urethra. Absolute sexual rest means the stallion is to be maintained in a location where he will not become sexually aroused.

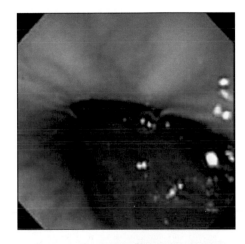

**Figure 12-16** Hemospermia: Blood clot in the urethra following semen collection.

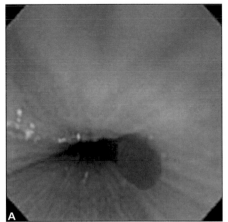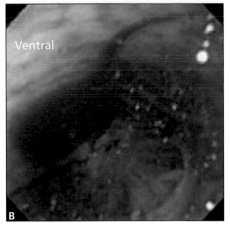

**Figure 12-17A,B** Panel A is an image of the penile urethra showing hematuria at urination. Panel B shows hematuria visible near the colliculus seminalis. The colliculus seminalis is visible in the lower right corner. The insufflation of air into the urethra during urination causes a backflow of urine and urine pooling due to urethral dilation. The bladder contains normal urine.

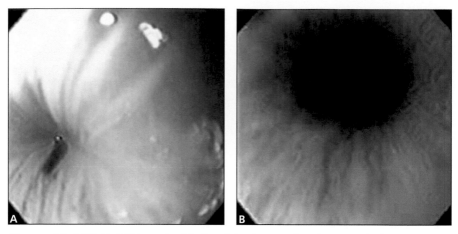

**Figure 12-18A,B** Mild urethral lesion (ulcer) – Panel A shows a shallow urethral ulcer in a stallion and Panel B is the same region of the urethra 3 months later.

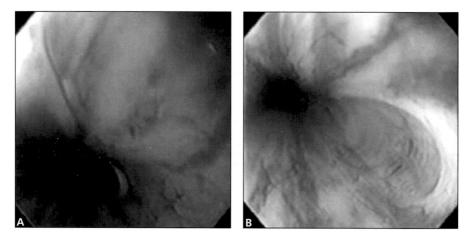

**Figure 12-19A,B** Moderate urethral lesion (tear) – Panel A shows a semicircular defect in the right wall of the urethra, panel B shows the same lesion at a higher level of insufflation.

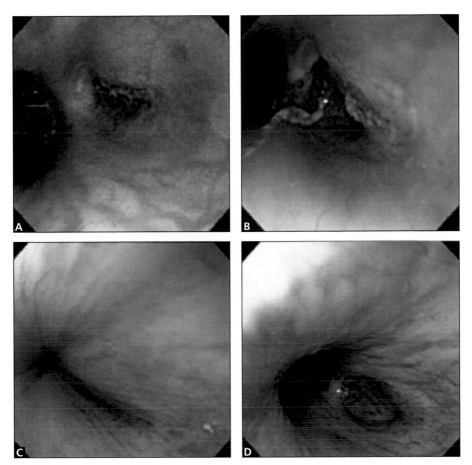

**Figure 12-20A-D** Severe urethral lesion (deep ulcerated urethral tear). Panel A shows a view of a fresh ulcerated urethral tear at the junction of the penile and pelvic portions of the urethra. Panel A shows the ulcerated urethral tear before urination, panel B shows the devitalized tissue in the ulcerated urethral tear after urination. Panels C-D show the same lesion 6 weeks after complete sexual rest with 2 levels of insufflation (Panel C low, Panel D moderate).

After the 3 week rest period, semen collection is performed and the lesion is re-evaluated using endoscopy. If the bleeding persists sexual rest is continued for 3 months. The evaluation process is repeated. If urethral bleeding continues past 3 months then an endoscopically guided subischial perineal urethrostomy is performed and left to granulate in. This allows the penile urethra to be rested from urine flow which appears to prevent healing of the urethra in some stallions.

✓ **Retrograde ejaculation** is an uncommon condition where the ejaculated sperm enter the bladder rather than being emitted from the penis. The problem arises in incomplete closure of the neck of the bladder, usually as a result of problems in the sympathetic nervous system. In these cases spermatozoa are recovered in the urine following ejaculation but are not emitted. There are no endoscopic abnormalities.

# Congenital Anomalies

✓ The majority of congenital anomalies in the reproductive tract of the intersex or stallion result in changes in appearance of the external genitalia. Phenotypic, gonadal and chromosomal sex, are typically investigated to determine the underlying cause.

✓ Embryonal remnanants such as a uterus masculinus, may sometimes be visualized. The opening to the uterus masculinus is usually located under the mound of the colliculus seminals.

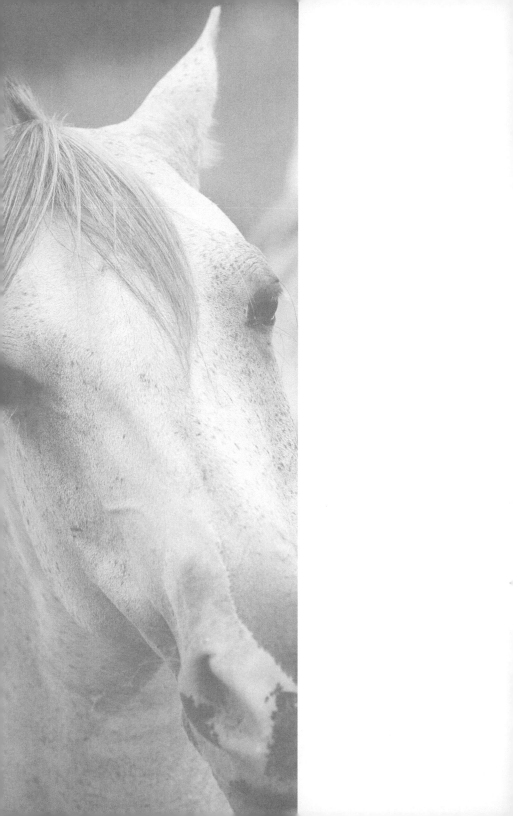

# Section 13

# Endoscopy of the Reproductive System of the Mare

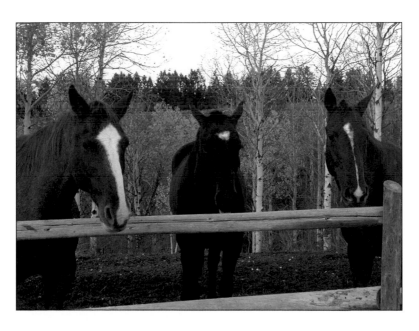

# Normal Anatomic Features

The structures of the mare's reproductive tract that may be viewed using endoscopy include: the vagina, vestibulovaginal fold, cervix, uterine body: bifurcation, uterine horn, and uterotubal papilla and ostium.

✓ The vagina in the mare is 18-23 cm long and 10-13 cm in diameter. The caudal portion of the vagina is sometimes referred to as the vestibule. The vestibule is formed by the genital folds of the urogenital sinus. The vesibule ends at the transverse fold, which is also called the vestibulovaginal sphincter. The hymen is present in this location. The hymen is a thin membrane like structure. It is the junction between the cranial vagina formed by the paramesonephric (Mullerian) duct system and the caudal vagina formed by the urogenital sinus. The hymen will not be visible in non-virgin mares. The urethra opens on the urethral tubercule on the ventral floor of the vagina at the vestibulovaginal fold.

✓ The cervix is located in the cranial vagina. The external os of the cervix protrudes into the vagina. The morphology of the cervix changes with the season and stage of the estrus cycle in the mare. In anestrus the cervix has little tone and may be seen to gape open slightly during a vaginal examination, and in the transition phase the cervical tone and prominence increase. During the breeding season the cervix is relaxed in estrus and edematous folds may obscure the opening, and in diestrus the cervix is non-edematous, tight and the opening prominent. There is a band of connective tissue located at 12 o'clock that extends from the wall of the vagina onto the cervix. This band is called the frenulum. It is a useful landmark when attempting to locate the cervix (Figure 13-1).

✓ The cervical canal in the mare may be easily penetrated using manual dilation. The internal os of the cervix opens into the body of the uterus. The interior of the cervical canal appears as a smooth surface during endoscopy (Figure 13-2).

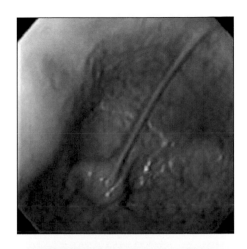

**Figure 13-1** Endoscopic view of the cranial vagina with the connective tissue frenulum visible running to the external cervical os of the cervix of a mare in estrus.

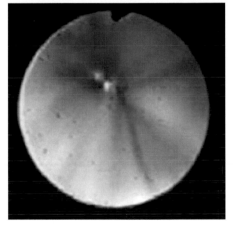

**Figure 13-2** Interior view of the smooth surface of the cervical canal.

✓ The uterus in the mare is Y shaped. The body of the uterus is about 20 cm in length. Greater than twelve longitudinal folds of endometrial mucosa form ridges which run from the body into the uterine horns. The entrance to the uterine horns from the body is called the bifurcation. The uterine horns are 15-20 cm in length and 4-7.5 cm in width. The longitudinal folds lead to the end of the uterine horn. The uterotubal ostium is located dorsally and eccentrically at the end of the horn. The ostium has the appearance of a papilla (Figure 13-9).

# Endoscopic Technique

✔ The endoscopic technique used to view the interior of the uterus is called hysteroscopy. Hysteroscopy is used often as an adjunct technique during a breeding soundness examination, and has specific applications for the diagnosis of certain conditions. Recently hysteroscopic insemination of low doses of semen have been used to obtain pregnancies.

♥ To prepare a mare for a hysteroscopic examination it is best to empty the rectum of manure. The perineum of the mare is cleansed, and the tail wrapped. Most mares are sedated intravenously using alpha-2 agonists, combined with butorphanol to minimize movement or any discomfort during the procedure. Sedation results in the mare leaning forward and dropping her head, so it is important that the mare is held in position near the back of the stocks using a chest rope for safety reasons and ensure that the full length of the endoscope is available for the examination. The mare should be observed while sedated so that she does not inadvertently close off her airway when her head drops, such as might occur if she rests her neck on the front gate of the stocks. The endoscopic equipment should be chemically sterilized and the disinfectant removed using alcohol and sterile water or saline. Generally 2 people are required to perform a hysteroscopic examination. An examiner passes the equipment through the vagina and cervix into different uterine locations, and an operator directs the tip of the endoscope when required. The examiner wears a clean rectal sleeve turned inside out with a sterile pair of surgical gloves over the rectal sleeve. The outer surface of the surgical glove, and sides but not the tip of the endoscope, are lubricated using a sterile methylcellulose lubricant. A one meter gastroscope, or videoendoscope is used. The examiner shields the end of the endoscope in their gloved hand and carries it forward to the cervix. The cervical canal is dilated by the examiner's finger and the endoscope is passed through the dilated cervical canal, so the tip just enters the uterine body. The cervix is then held closed around the endoscope and the uterus is insufflated. Typically with fully functional endoscopic equipment, complete uterine insufflation should take less than 20 seconds. If the uterus is not readily insufflating an external insufflation source way be used. A sterile catheter is attached to a flow regulator connected to a pressurized tank of room air, or nitrous oxide, and the other end is passed down the biopsy channel of the endoscope. The gas flow is turned on and the uterus is insufflated. Excess uterine insufflation results in gas being released through the cervix. The insufflated state of the uterus is maintained using intermittent air flow during the hysteroscopic examination.

# The Normal Endometrium

✓ The normal endometrium of the mare is pale pink and appears to have a homogenous texture. The uterus should be evaluated for colour, texture, the presence of discharge, foreign matter, endometrial cysts, lymphatic cysts, and presence of adhesions.

In estrus, there will be glistening mucus present on the surface of the endometrium and endometrial edema will be prominent. The folds of the uterus will be visibly edematous (Figures 13-3 through 13-8, Figure 13-10).

♥ The process of uterine involution in the mare is rapid, and in an uncomplicated foaling the uterus of the mare will be one and half times its non-pregnant size by 12 hours post-partum. The normal lochia of the mare is low volume, thick and reddish in color (Figure 13-11).

☷ The uterine body typically is situated in the pelvis, with the opening to the uterine horns located cranioventrally. The cranioventral curve must to followed to atraumatically enter and evaluate the uterine horns. Minimal manipulation of the tip of the endoscope is used to pass the endoscope into the uterine horns. The examiner, using their hand in the mare's vagina and another on the endoscope, feeds and directs the endoscope into the uterine horns. Once a uterine horn has been entered the directional turning knobs of the endoscope may be locked and the tip of the scope directed using fine manipulation as needed.

☷ Samples such as swabs, or biopsies may be obtained through the biopsy port of the endoscope. Once the entire contents of the uterus has been viewed, the air flow is turned off and the biopsy portal opened to allow the gas to be released from the uterus. Transrectal palpation may be used to encourage the emptying of air. It is important to rinse and clean the equipment following each procedure to keep the endoscope functional and to reduce the potential for mechanical transfer of pathogens between patients. Iatrogenic infection is a risk of the procedure.

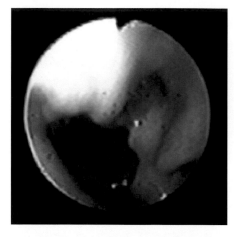

**Figure 13-3** Partially insufflated uterine body showing endometrial folds.

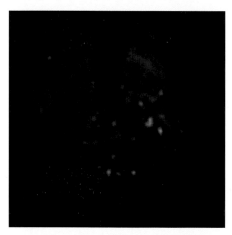

**Figure 13-4** Hysteroscopic view of the uterine body looking toward the internal cervical os. The view is obtained by turning the endoscope back on itself.

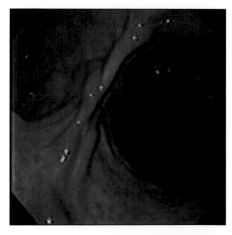

**Figure 13-5** Hysteroscopic view of the bifurcation of the uterus of an estrous mare.

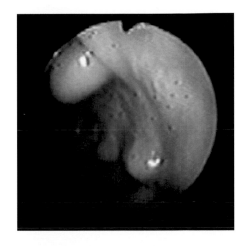

**Figure 13-6** Hysteroscopic view of endometrial folds.

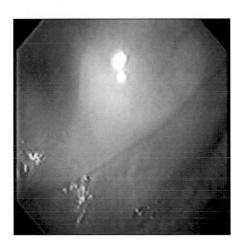

**Figure 13-7** Hysteroscopic view of edematous endometrial folds of an estrous mare.

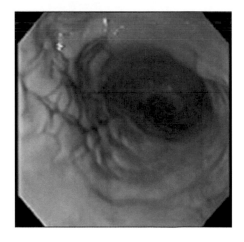

**Figure 13-8** Hysteroscopic view of a uterine horn.

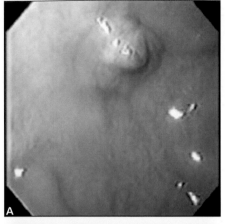

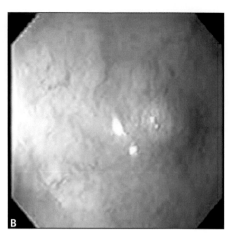

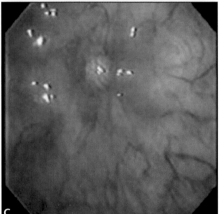

**Figure 13-9A-C** Hysteroscopic views of the end of the uterine horn at the uterotubal junction. The uterotubal papilla are somewhat variable in their external morphology; the papilla from 3 different estrous mares are shown in each panel as a small, lighter-coloured raised area.

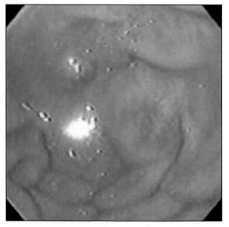

**Figure 13-10** Hysteroscopic view of a healthy endometrium in an estrous mare.

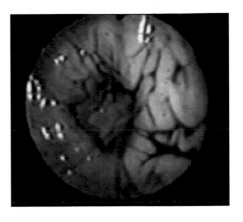

**Figure 13-11** Hysteroscopic image of a mare's post-partum uterus showing lochia and large number of endometrial folds at the entrance to a uterine horn.

# Endometrial Biopsy

✓ Iatrogenic bleeding at the site of an endometrial biopsy is a normal finding. Uterine biopsies where large strips of tissue come away, when the instrument is dull, or when biopsies are taken from mares with fibrotic endometrial changes tend to bleed more excessively. The presence of bleeding after a biopsy procedure is performed is a normal finding and should be taken into account when performing a hysteroscopic procedure after a biopsy (Figure 13-12).

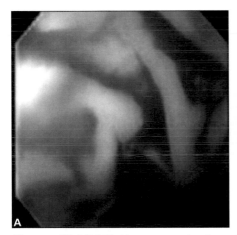
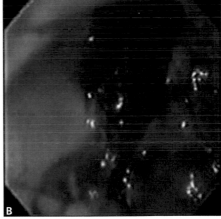

**Figure 13-12A,B** Hysteroscopic view of the endometrium following a uterine biopsy procedure. Panel (A) shows fresh blood trapped in the endometrial folds, while panel (B) shows a blood clot adherent to the site of the biopsy.

# Hysteroscopic Cannulation and Insemination

♥ A hysteroscopic approach was developed to cannulate the uterotubal ostium. In the normal mare the volume of the uterine tube is 300 microliters, and small volumes may be injected into the uterine tube by cannulating the utero-tubal ostium (Figure 13-13). In a mare with patent uterine tubes the injection will occur with some pressure and may be used as a means of evaluating tubal patency, however the procedure is technically difficult.

♥ Hysteroscopic insemination is a low dose insemination technology. A reduced number and minute insemination volume are used in this technique. The side where the dominant follicle is located is determined. The endoscope is directed up the uterine horn ipsilateral to the dominant follicle. A small catheter is passed through the biopsy channel of the endoscope and advanced so it touches the uterotubal papilla. The inseminate is then injected onto the surface of the papilla. This insemination technique has been successful with fresh, frozen, and sex-selected spermatozoa (Figure 13-14).

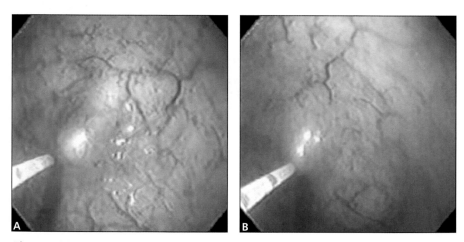

**Figure 13-13A,B** The top panel (A) shows the approach to the uterotubal papilla and the bottom panel (B) is a hysteroscopic view of a cannulation of the uterotubal ostium.

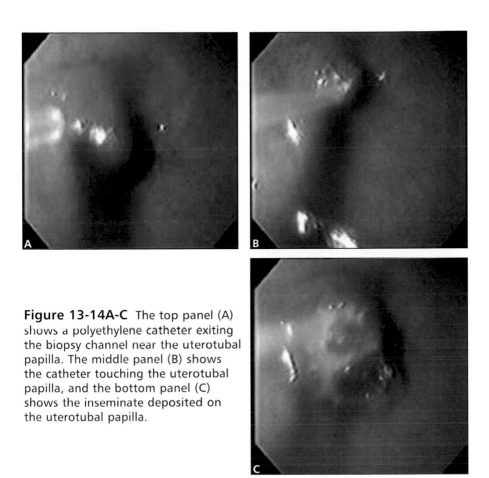

**Figure 13-14A-C** The top panel (A) shows a polyethylene catheter exiting the biopsy channel near the uterotubal papilla. The middle panel (B) shows the catheter touching the uterotubal papilla, and the bottom panel (C) shows the inseminate deposited on the uterotubal papilla.

# Pathologic Conditions of the Vagina

## Urovagina

♥ Urovagina is a condition where urine accumulates in the vagina and causes a chemical inflammation. A predisposing factor for urovagina is pneumovagina. Pneumovagina is caused by poor perineal conformation and may occur post–foaling due to stretching of the reproductive tract, and the opening of Caslick for foaling in mares with poor perineal conformation. The urine should be removed from the vagina of the mare using a speculum or cotton before a hysteroscopic examination is performed. Persistent urovagina may be due to a dysfunction or injury to the bladder, or urethra, or may be due to an ectopic ureter.

# Vaginal Hematoma and Abscesses

✓ Vaginal hematomas occur primarily as a result of an injury during foaling. Hematomas may become secondarily infected. The depth of an abscess may sometimes be determined using an endoscope.

# Vaginal Lacerations

✓ Vaginal lacerations may accompany foaling or breeding. Certain stallions are known to cause vaginal injuries to mares and these stallions are used for breeding using artificial insemination or by using a breeding roll to prevent deep penile penetration. The extent of the vaginal laceration or injury may be explored using endoscopy.

# Varicose Veins

✓ Varicose veins are tortuous venous structures that may bleed during pregnancy. They are more common in older mares. A dry vagina resulting from pneumovagina predisposes to the varicose veins becoming fragile and bleeding. The veins are usually difficult to locate and frequently are found dorsally at the vestibulo-vaginal junction. Endoscopy may be used to help locate the offending bleeding vessels. A Caslick may solve the mare's problem by eliminating the vaginal dryness after a week or more as the vaginal environment becomes restored to a moister state, or the vessels may need to be ligated, cauterized or injected with a sclerosing solution.

# Vaginal Fusion

♥ Vaginal fusion is typically diagnosed following severe foaling trauma or a difficult dystocia. Miniature horses due to their small size, and subsequent difficulty in fixing their obstetrical problems, are prone to this foaling complication. In cases of vaginal fusion the mucosa is injured and inflamed resulting in the sides of the vagina literally adhering and fusing together. Urination keeps a small passageway open from the bladder to the vulva. Endoscopy of the narrow channel may be used to assess the extent of the vaginal fusion (Figure 13-15).

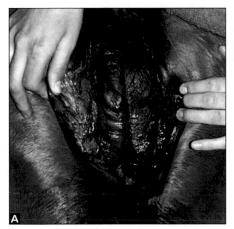

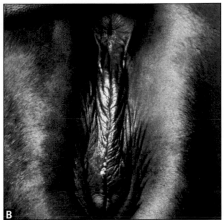

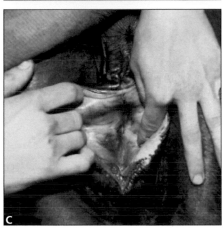

**Figure 13-15A-C** The top panel (A) shows the severely traumatized vulva of a mare subsequent to a dystocia where the contracted forelimbs of her foal missed the vulvar opening and ruptured through each side of the vulva. Massive vulvovaginitis and secondary peritonitis resulted. The mare survived and Panel (B) shows the mare's vulva 6 months later. A vaginal exam revealed that the vagina was fused. Panel (C) shows the opening that allowed the passage of urine. Endoscopy of the opening revealed that all but 10 cm of the vagina near the cervix, were fused together.

# Pathologic Conditions of the Cervix

## Cervical Lacerations

✓ Cervical lacerations typically occur as a consequence of a foaling injury. Endoscopy may be used to evaluate the extent of the injury. Lacerations that involve only the external cervical os carry a better prognosis than injuries that penetrate the cervical canal.

## Cervical Adhesions

♥ Foaling injuries or injuries to the cervix during fetotomy procedures may result in significant cervicitis that results in the formation of transluminal adhesions. Transluminal cervical adhesions are associated with the development of pyometra in mares.

# Pathologic Conditions of the Uterus

♥ The endometrium of subfertile mares, with a significant degree of lymphstasis, has a reticular pattern. These subfertile mares are prone to intrauterine fluid accumulation during breeding and have a defect in uterine contractility (Figure 13-16).

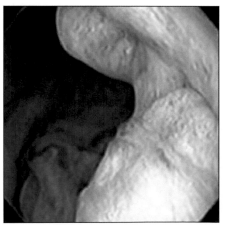

**Figure 13-16** A hysteroscopic view of a subfertile mare's endometrium with lymphstasis, showing a reticular rather than homogenous endometrial pattern.

# Endometritis

⚷ Acute uterine inflammation associated with endometritis may be identified in mares. In mares physiologic processes such as breeding, or foaling cause only transient short lived inflammation. Persistent inflammation of the endometrium is associated with lower fertility and uterine subinvolution in foaling mares. Acute endometritis is characterized by the presence of cloudy, free intrauterine fluid, that is neutrophil laden. A vaginal discharge may also be evident. Uterine discharge is usually caused by bacterial infection, should be evaluated using cytology and culture. In post partum mares, high volume, foul smelling watery uterine discharge is associated with post-foaling endometritis. Normal lochia is thick and low volume.

# Endometrial, Glandular and Lymphatic Cysts

⚷ Endometrial cysts are small structures usually less than 1mm in diameter. Endometrial lymphatic cysts vary in size and number, and may be identified as solitary cysts or clusters (Figure 13-17). They may be larger than 6 cm in diameter (Figure 13-18). Lymphatic cysts may have compartments, or may be found in clusters. They may or may not be spherical like embryos. Structures such as endometrial cysts or endometrial lymphatic cysts by themselves are not clinically significant. A few cysts of either type are not associated with fertility problems in mares. Cysts may be present in subfertile and fertile mares.

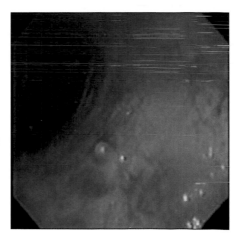

**Figure 13-17** This is a hysteroscopic view of the uterus showing a small round endometrial cyst. Endometrial cysts correspond histologically to dilated endometrial glands and contain glandular secretions.

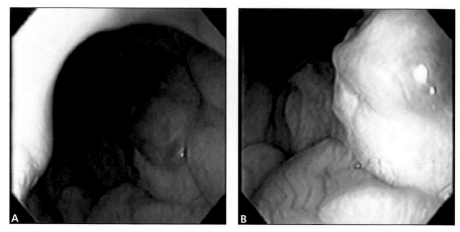

**Figure 13-18A,B** Shown are 2 hysteroscopic views of a uterine lymphatic cyst. In panel (A) the lymphatic cyst is the bluish opaque structure in the top right portion of the field, the same cyst is shown in a closer view in panel (B).

Larger lymphatic cysts may be confused with embryos during an ultrasound examination, or result in the diagnosis of a twin pregnancy, when a cyst and an embryo are present. It is clinically important to note the location and size of cysts in the uterus. Cysts grow very slowly, may be found year after year, and unlike embryos, do not develop heart beats. For this reason if there is no previous examination history a mare should not be diagnosed in foal until an embryo with a heart beat is identified, or prior to that time a structure "compatible with an embryonic vesicle" should be recorded.

✔ Occasionally a lymphatic cyst is deemed to be large enough to interfere with embryonic migration or sperm transport. The lymphatic cyst may be ruptured using a laser through a hysteroscopic approach, and then removed at its base (Figure 13-19).

♥ Rarely an aembryonic vesicle forms where no embryonic body is identified. These pregnancies are self limiting and are eventually spontaneously eliminated. The mare may be returned to estrus using prostaglandin by 35 days but after that time endometrial cups form and prevent the mare from coming back into heat for months.

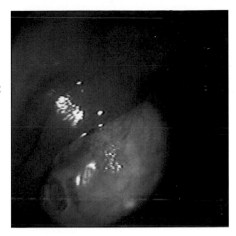

**Figure 13-19** Shown is a hysteroscopic image of cyst where light from a laser is visible behind a lymphatic cyst. A laser induced injury is present as an oval in the left side of the lymphatic cyst.

# Pyometra

Pyometra is a condition in which the uterus fills with pus. True pyometra in a mare usually involves a cervical injury that mechanically interferes with emptying of the uterus. The endometrium is often diseased as well such that it looses its ability to secrete prostaglandin, resulting in retained luteal tissue and prolonged diestrous periods. The diseased endometrium looses its normal smooth appearance (Figure 13-20). The chronic retention of pus in the mare's uterus may result in mild anemia or no systemic change in the blood count. The fluid may or may not grow bacteria when cultured.

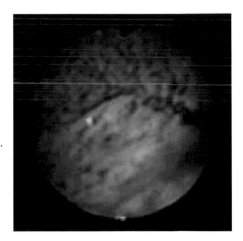

**Figure 13-20** Hysteroscopic view of the damaged endometrium of a mare that developed a pyometra following a fetotomy that caused cervical adhesions.

# Persistent Endometrial Cups

✓ Persistent endometrial cups are a rare finding in mares that fail to establish normal estrus cycles post foaling. These mares have persistently high levels of eCG. There is a failure of the endometrial cup tissue to regress. The cup tissue may be visualized using endoscopy.

# Transluminal Adhesions

✓ Transluminal uterine adhesion may result due to trauma and inflammation following dystocia, hysterotomy, or intrauterine infusion of caustic materials (Figure 13-21).

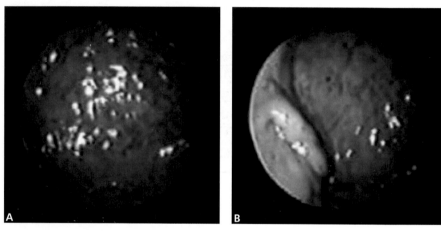

**Figure 13-21A,B** This is a hysteroscopic view of a mare with a damaged endometrium. Panel (A) shows ulcerated areas. Panel (B) shows a uterine adhesion that involves a uterine fold. The adhesion is causing the uterine fold to take a right angle turn, which is visible on the left side of the image.

# Tumors of the Uterus and Cervix

☞ The most common cervical and uterine tumor is a leiomyoma (Figures 13-22 and 13-23). These are slow growing tumors that form from the proliferation of cells that resemble smooth muscle. If other tissue elements are more active, or the tumor is more invasive, the tumor may be called a fibroleiomyoma, or leiomyosarcoma. Small tumors of this classification may be followed and may not interfere with fertility. Larger tumors may obstruct the uterine lumen, become necrotic on the surface as they outgrow their blood supply, and interfere with fertility. This type of tumour is removed using a surgical approach. A mare must have 70% of her uterus remaining following surgery for her to recognize the presence of the embryo and carry her own pregnancy to term. Uterine adenocarcinomas have also been reported and result in significant tissue damage, and frequent uterine discharge. The differential diagnoses of a mass in the uterine wall includes tumor, and intramural hematoma formation. Intramural hematomas occur following foaling, and generally slowly resolve over time.

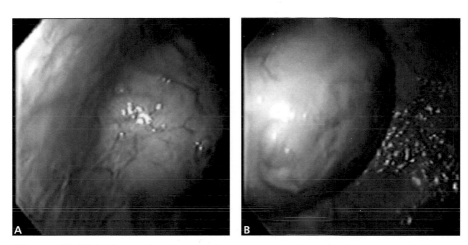

**Figure 13-22A,B** Panel A shows a hysteroscopic view of a leiomyoma bulging into the interior of a uterine horn. Panel B is another view of the tumour that shows the yellow necrotic surface and a region where the tumour is breaching the endometrium.

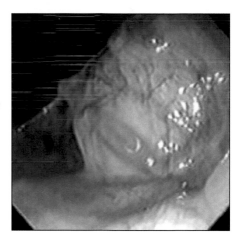

**Figure 13-23** A hysteroscopic view of a uterine leiomyoma in the uterine body of a mare.

# Foreign Bodies

✓ Foreign bodies in the mare's uterus often involve broken parts of culture swabs including parts of the rod and the sample tip. The broken ends of culture swabs are often retrieved manually by dilating the cervix and retrieving the missing piece, or by using uterine lavage to flush out the pieces. In some cases implements such as endoscopic biopsy tools, or a biopsy forcep may be used to dislodge a foreign body that is embedded or trapped in the endometrium. A tool may be used to drag the piece near the cervix for retrieval (Figure 13-24).

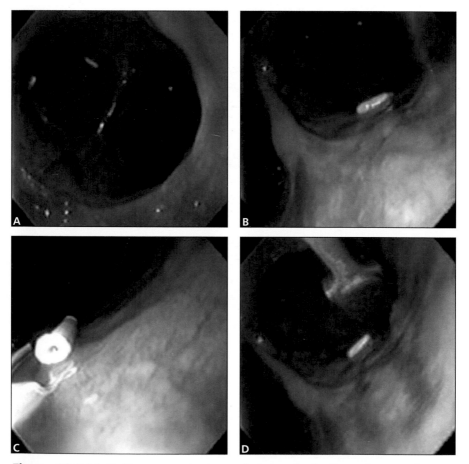

**Figure 13-24A-D** Hysteroscopic views of pieces of a broken culture swab retained in mare's uterus. The lower panel (D) shows a biopsy instrument being used to help move the foreign object to a location near the cervix so that it may be manually retrieved.

# Fetal Maceration or Mummification

✓ Occasionally a fetus dies and the mummified or macerated bones are retained in the mare's uterus. The bones may be adherent to the endometrium and require manipulations such as bringing the mare into heat and using manual cervical dilation or use of tools through the endoscope's biopsy port to dislodge them.

# Uterine Lacerations

♥ The uterus of the mare may be injured during foaling. Full thickness lacerations of the dorsal portion of the uterine horn are the most common injury. This may result in significant abdominal contamination and peritonitis. These mares present as depressed post-partum mares. Some advocate the use of hysteroscopy to help visualize the tear to confirm the diagnosis. The post-partum uterus is difficult to insufflate due to its large volume, large cervix and excessive endometrial folds. A laceration further increases the difficulty in achieving good insufflation.

# Retained Fetal Membranes

⚷ Mares may retain all or part of their fetal membranes. Retention of the tip of the non-pregnancy horn is the most common problem. This is why foaling attendants should evaluate the fetal membranes to determine if all of it has been delivered. Mares following Cesarian section may have the fetal membranes inadvertently tacked into the hysterotomy closure. Mares with retained fetal membranes usually show clinical signs (endotoxemia, laminitis) by 12-24 hours post partum. Subinvolution of the uterus, foul-smelling fluid discharge, echogenic material in the uterus are all indications of retained fetal membranes. Hysteroscopy is sometimes used to evaluate an incision area in a post foaling mare, or to identify the location of a piece of the fetal membranes.

# Congenital Abnormalities

♥ Congenital abnormalities of the vagina, cervix and uterus in the mare have been reported. Imperforate hymens have been reported, and mucoid material may be present behind the septum. In athletic mares the hymen may bulge out through the vulva during exercise. A paramesonephric duct remnant (persistent mullerian) remnant in the mare forms a longitudinal septum like a division of the vagina. Cervical aplasia has also been reported. A double cervix either communicating or not communicating with a uterus, or to separate uterine horns has been reported. Uterus unicornis, and uterus bicollis have been reported in the mare. These conditions are frequently investigated using hysteroscopy to confirm the nature of the problem. Mares with the 63XO genotype have a small flaccid cervix and uterus. Ectopic ureters that empty into the vagina have also been reported.

# Pathologic Conditions of the Rectum

## Rectal Stricture

💣 Mares that strain excessively during a dystocia, particularly as a result of excessive traction on their fetuses, may prolapse their rectum and develop rectal injuries. The mesocolic artery in the mare is the main blood supply to the caudal rectum. Prolapse of the rectum may result in rupture or damage to this artery with subsequent devitalization and necrosis of the rectum. The examiner may not be able to perform a rectal examination due to a stricture of the devitalized tissue. The rectum may be evaluated by placing a clear speculum into the rectum, a Caslick type speculum or through endoscopy. A yellowish necrotic area may be seen in the rectum when this injury occurs.

## Rectal Tears

♥ Rectal tears may occur as a consequence of foaling. Small bowel or small intestine often prolapse through these rectal tears. Iatrogenic rectal tears are a major cause of professional liability claims. Rectal injury is a well recognized risk of rectal examination. The overall risk of injury is low, but the consequences of a full-thickness rectal injury are high. If a popping or yielding sensation is felt during a rectal examination, or blood is found on the examiner's rectal sleeve following the examination, it should trigger further investigation. Bleeding may be caused by rectal mucosal irritation, mucosal injury, mucosal and submucosal injury and full-thickness injuries. Speculum examination of the rectum, palpation of the lesion, and endoscopy are often used to determine if a rectal injury extends from the submucosa into the abdomen. Endoscopy is particularly useful in cases where the lesion dissects away from the rectal luminal injury. Visualization of bowel is confirmation of a full thickness injury.

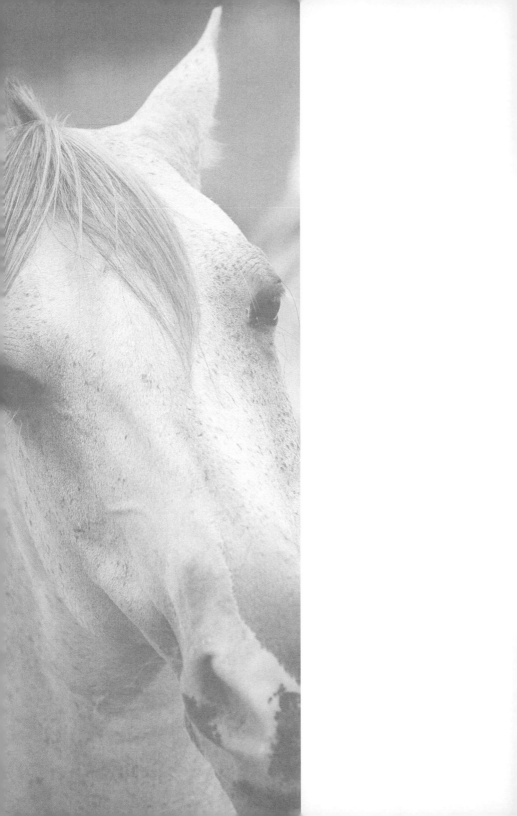

# Section 14

# Arthroscopy

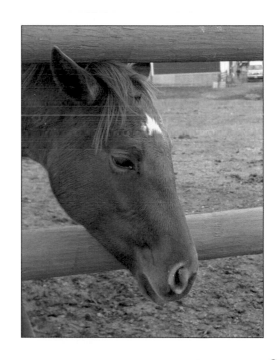

# Introduction

✓ Arthroscopy and tenoscopy have become the major joint/tendon sheath exploration and treatment methods of both human and veterinary surgery.

✓ Arthroscopy and laparoscopic surgery take the need for three-dimensional perception to an advanced level and requires significant practice to perfect.

✓ Benefits over arthrotomy and open approaches to the tendon sheaths include:

- Lower patient morbidity.
- Reduced convalescent time.
- Improved post-operative performance.
- Better intra-operative visualization of intra-articular lesions (in the majority of cases).

# Instrumentation

Basic instrumentation necessary for arthroscopic surgery includes: (Figures 14-1 and 14-2).

- A 4 mm arthroscope (30° lens angle).
- Cannula with stopcock.
- Blunt and sharp obturators for joint entry.
- A light source (fibreoptic).
- Videocamera and viewing monitor.
- Fluid irrigation system and an egress cannula.

Hand instruments commonly used include:

- Blunt probe.
- Arthroscopic knife.
- Ferris-Smith and ethmoid rongeurs.
- Elevators and curette.
- +/– Synovial resector (a motorized instrument characterized by a rotating blade contained in a sheath with a side-opening allowing synovial membrane to be trapped, cut and evacuated from the joint).

✓ All equipment should be sterilized and be used observing aseptic technique at all times.

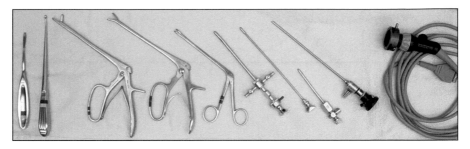

**Figure 14-1** From left to right: Periosteal elevator, Curette, straight Ferris-Smith rongeurs, angled Ferris-Smith rongeurs, ethmoid forceps, cannula with blunt obturator, sharp obturator, egress cannula, 30 degree Wolf arthroscope, videocamera.

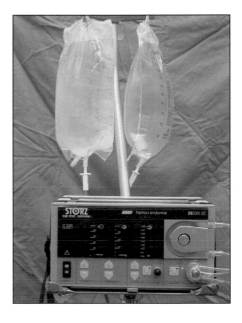

**Figure 14-2** Storz arthroscopic fluid pump with attached fluid.

# Pre- & Post-Surgical Considerations

✓ Preoperative treatment with potassium penicillin and phenylbutazone.

✓ Post-operative intra-articular administration of 200 mg gentamicin and an appropriate dose of bupivicaine.

✓ Skin closure using a 2-0 non-absorbable suture in a cruciate pattern. No attempt is made to close the joint capsule, in most cases.

✓ Extensive stifle surgery may warrant consideration of epidural analgesia.

♥ Monitoring post-operative fecal production is important to prevent the development of large colon impaction which may be a result of a pain-induced ileus.

# Technique Hints

✓ Skin incisions for carpal and tibiotarsal joint arthroscopy are made, avoiding the tendon sheaths and saphenous vein respectively, prior to joint distention.

✓ Joint expansion with isotonic solutions prior to arthroscope placement (NOT femorotibial joints).

✓ Confirmation of joint entry is obtained prior to joint distention in femorotibial arthroscopy.

Joint distention results in the capsule being presented immediately under skin incisions to allow puncture using a scalpel blade or sharp obturator / cannula combination.

Failure to inflate the joint sufficiently may predispose the operator to inadvertent subcutaneous tissue placement of the arthroscope.

✓ Initial skin incision for the arthroscope portal using a #15 blade.

♥ Slightly larger than that made through the joint capsule to limit subcutaneous fluid pooling in the event of fluid extravasation during surgery.

♥ Capsule incision made with a #11 blade.

A single stab incision is made perpendicular to the joint capsule.

The blade is removed, rotated 180 degrees, and the stabbing motion repeated.

No rocking motion of the blade is made.

❤ Arthroscope portal is placed contralateral to the region of interest in most cases.

✓ Instrument portals are placed ipselateral and in most cases the exact positioning is determined using a spinal needle prior to skin incision.

# Common Pathological Conditions

❤ Sepsis: Usually characterized by severe (can be non-weight bearing) lameness, joint effusion and pyrexia. In some cases (especially coffin and pastern joints) peri-articular edema. Intra-articular pathology includes synovial hyperemia, edema, fibrin accumulation and in some cases osteochondral fragments. The most common etiological agents include *Staphylococcus aureus* (post-surgery), *Streptococcus spp.* and *Pseudomonas spp.*

✓ Osteochondrosis: A failure of endochondral ossification which has certain predilection sites within a specific joint e.g.: the distal intermediate ridge of the tibia (DIRT) within the hock. When a fissured cartilage flap has a degree of calcification but is still attached at one edge it can be termed osteochondrosis dissecans (OCD). Cystic lesions (e.g.: medial femoral condyles) have been identified as a manifestation of osteochondrosis however there is some debate as to whether this is accurate. Similar lesions have been created traumatically in experimental situations in which the subchondral plate is damaged in addition to the overlying cartilage.

✓ Osteochondral Fragmentation: Chip fractures (such as proximal P1 fractures) that include cartilage overlying bone can be termed osteochondral fragments and can include those fragments originating from osteochondrosis lesions as well as traumatic fractures.

✓ Other common conditions include foreign body penetration and soft tissue injuries (ligaments-collateral and cruciate ligaments as well as meniscal damage).

# Specific Joints (Approaches and Pathology)

## Coffin Joint

### (Distal Interphalangeal Joint)

### Dorsal Approach

✓ Recumbency: Dorsal or Lateral.

✓ Portal Placement: 3 cm proximal to the coronary band, immediately abaxial to the common/long digital extensor tendon (3 cm abaxial to the midline) (Figure 14-3).

✓ Entrance Angle: Towards distal P2, and an angle across the joint to go under the extensor tendon.

♥ Common Mistakes:

- Inappropriate angle and soft tissue penetrance.
- Failure to use a tourniquet.
  - Standard or Eshmark for extensor process fracture removal significantly improves visualization.

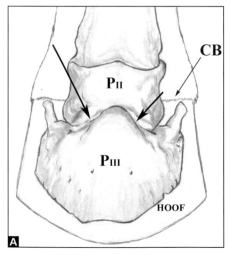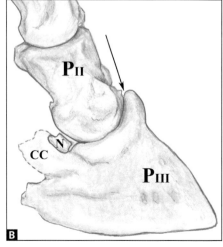

**Figure 14-3A,B** Dorsal (A) and lateral (B) anatomical drawings indicating the correct position and angle of the arthroscope during examination of the coffin joint (arrows). (PI-Proximal phalanx, PII-Second phalanx, PIII-Third phalanx (coffin bone), CB – coronary band, N-Navicular bone, CC – Colateral Cartilages of the coffin bone).

✓ Normal Anatomy:

- Extensor process of P3.
- Distal condyles of P2.
- Collateral ligaments of the coffin joint (Figure 14-4).

♥ Pathological Processes:

- Extensor process fractures (traumatic).
- Extensor process fractures (possible osteochondrosis) (Figures 14-5 through 14-7).
- P3 cysts.
- Sepsis.

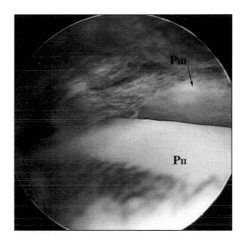

**Figure 14-4** Lateral compartment of distal interphalangeal joint: Third (P$_{III}$) and second (P$_{II}$) phalanges.

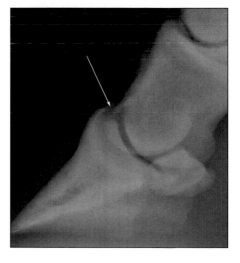

**Figure 14-5** Traumatic extensor process fracture in a yearling horse.

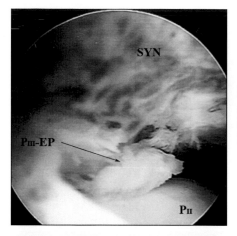

**Figure 14-6** Dorsolateral to distomedial view within the coffin joint. Extensor process fracture of P3 ($P_{III}$ – EP), $P_{II}$ – Second phalanx, SYN – synovium.

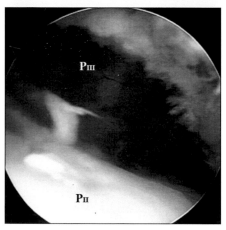

**Figure 14-7** Distal Interphalangeal joint (dorsoproximal to dorsodistal view): Debrided fracture bed ($P_{III}$) distal condyle of P2 ($P_{II}$).

# Palmar / Plantar Approach

✓ Recumbency: Dorsal or Lateral.

✓ Portal Placement: 2 cm proximal to the heel bulbs, immediately axial to the collateral cartilages of P3 and the neurovascular bundle, and abaxial to the flexor tendon sheath (Figure 14-8).

✓ Entrance Angle: As steep as possible, passing immediately palmar / plantar to the distal condyle of P2, aiming towards the point of the frog.

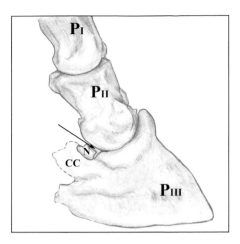

**Figure 14-8** Anatomical drawing indicating the correct position and angle of the arthroscope during examination of the palmar / plantar coffin joint (arrow). ($P_I$ – Proximal phalanx, $P_{II}$ – Second phalanx, $P_{III}$ – Third phalanx (coffin bone), N-Navicular bone, CC – Colateral Cartilages of the coffin bone).

♥ Common Mistakes:
  • Entrance into the navicular bursa.
  • Flexor tendon sheath or soft tissue penetrance.

✓ Normal Anatomy:
  • Distal condyles of P2 (Figure 14-9).
  • Navicular bone (Figure 14-10).
  • Palmar / plantar aspect of P3 (Figure 14-11).
  • Collateral ligaments of the navicular bone (Figure 14-12).

♥ Pathological Processes:
  • Collateral ligament damage.
  • Navicular bone fracture.
  • Sepsis.

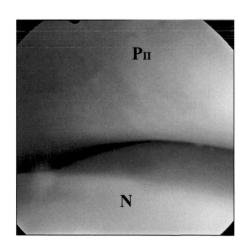

**Figure 14-9** The palmar approach to the coffin joint. Distal second phalanx ($P_{II}$) and the navicular bones (N) can be seen.

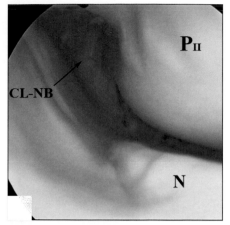

**Figure 14-10** Lateral view using the palmar approach. Distal second phalanx ($P_{II}$) and the navicular bones (N) can be seen as well as the collateral ligament of the navicular bone (CL-NB).

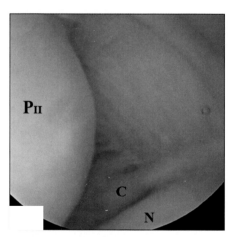

**Figure 14-11** Palmaroproximal to Palmarodistal view of the coffin joint. Distal second phalanx ($P_{II}$), navicular bone (N) and coffin bone (C).

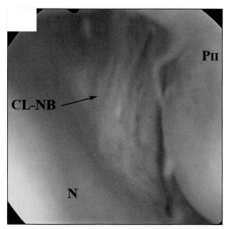

**Figure 14-12** Looking medially the palmar approach. Distal second phalanx ($P_{II}$) and the navicular bones (N) can be seen as well as the collateral ligament of the navicular bone (CL-NB).

# Pastern Joint
## (Proximal Interphalangeal Joint)
## Dorsal Approach
✓ Recumbency: Lateral.

✓ Portal Placement: Immediately dorsal to distal P2, underneath the extensor tendons, on a line 2 to 3 cm proximal to the level of the distal condyles of P2 (Figure 14-13).

✓ Entrance Angle: In a frontal plane, across the face of the joint.

♥ Common Mistakes:
  • Placing the portals too high, resulting in limited views of the dorsal joint space.

✓ Normal Anatomy:
  • Joint capsule
  • Distal P1
  • Proximal P2 (Figure 14-14)

♥ Pathological Processes:
  • Degenerative joint disease
  • Osteochondral chip fragments
  • Sepsis

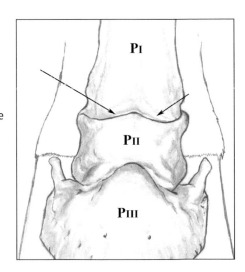

Figure 14-13 Anatomical drawing indicating the correct position and angle of the arthroscope during examination of the pastern joint (arrows). (P$_I$ – Proximal phalanx, P$_{II}$ – Second phalanx, P$_{III}$ – Third phalanx (coffin bone).

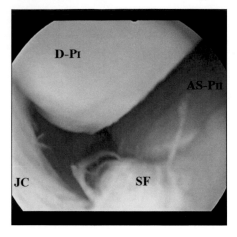

**Figure 14-14** Distal proximal phalanx (D-P$_I$), Proximal second phalanx and articular surface (AS-P$_{II}$), SF – Synovial frond and JC – Joint capsule.

# Palmar / Plantar Approach

✓ Recumbency: Lateral.

✓ Portal Placement: 2 to 3 cm proximal to the distal condyles of P2, in the "V" formed by the insertion of the superficial digital flexor tendon (Figure 14-15).

✓ Entrance Angle: Distally and axially.

✓ Normal Anatomy:

- Joint capsule
- Distal P1
- Proximal P2.

♥ Pathological Processes:

- Rare.
- OC fragments

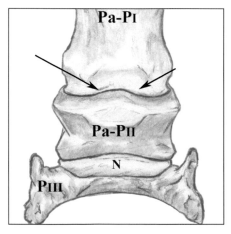

**Figure 14-15** Anatomical drawing indicating the correct position and angle of the arthroscope during examination of the palmar / plantar pastern joint (arrows). (Pa-P$_I$ – Palmar aspect of proximal phalanx, Pa-P$_{II}$ – Palmar aspect of second phalanx, P$_{III}$ – Third phalanx (coffin bone), N – Navicular bone).

# Fetlock Joint

## (Metacarpo / Tarso Phalangeal Joint)

✓ Recumbency: Dorsal or Lateral.

## Dorsal Approach

✓ Portal Placement: Proximolaterally or proximomedially in the dorsal joint pouch (Figure 14-16).

✓ Entrance Angle: Initially perpendicular to the skin incision and then parallel to the joint surface to avoid damage to the articular cartilage, on the sagittal ridge of distal MCIII.

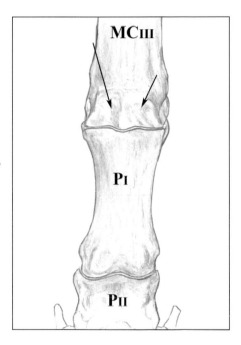

**Figure 14-16** Anatomical drawing indicating the correct position and angle of the arthroscope during examination of the dorsal aspect of the fetlock joint (arrows). MC$_{III}$ – Third metacarpal / tarsal bone (cannon bone), P$_I$ – Proximal phalanx, P$_{II}$ – Second phalanx.

♥ Common Mistakes:
- Subcutaneous placement of the cannula.
- Iatrogenic MC/MTIII sagittal ridge trauma.

✓ Normal Anatomy: (Figures 14-17 through 14-19)
- Sagittal ridge of MCIII.
- Medial and lateral condyles of MCIII.
- Proximo-medial and lateral dorsal P1.
- Dorsal synovial pad of fetlock joint.

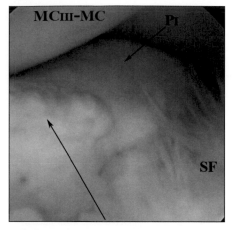

**Figure 14-17** Latero-Medial View: Medial condyle of distal MCIII ($MC_{III}$ – MC), proximal first phalanx ($P_I$), synovial fronds (SF) and irregular margin to dorsal $P_I$ (arrow).

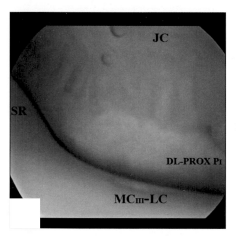

**Figure 14-18** Proximo-Distal View: Distal lateral condyle MCIII ($MC_{III}$-LC), Sagittal ridge (SR), Dorsolateral proximal P1 (DL-PROX $P_I$) and joint capsule (JC).

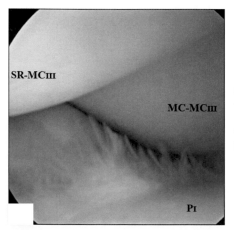

**Figure 14-19** DorsoLateral to PalmaroMedial View: Sagittal ridge of MCIII (SR-$MC_{III}$), Medial condyle MCIII (MC-$MC_{III}$), articular surface of proximal phalanx ($P_I$).

♥ Pathological Processes:
- Osteochondral fragments.
  - Osteochondrosis–Sagittal ridge MCIII.
  - Proximomedial P1 chip fractures (Figure14-20).
- Foreign Body.
- Synovial hyperplasia.
- Sepsis.

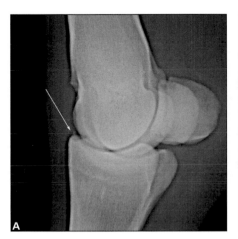
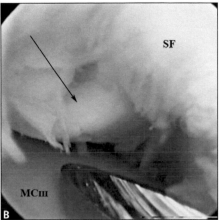

**Figure 14-20A,B** A: Digital radiograph of a yearling horse with a proximal dorsomedial P1 OC fragment. B: Intra-operative arthroscopic view of the same horse. Distal cannon bone (MC$_{III}$), synovial fronds (SF) and osteochondral fragment proximal P1 (arrow).

# Palmar / Plantar Approach

✓ Portal Placement: Proximally in the palmar / plantar fetlock joint pouch (Figure 14-21).

✓ Entrance Angle: Distally and axially, with the joint in moderate flexion to enable the arthroscope to pass between the condyles of MC$_{III}$ and the sesamoid bones.

✓ Normal Anatomy: (Figures 14-22 through 14-26)
- Medial and Lateral sesamoid bones.
- Intersesamoidean ligament.
- Mid-sagittal ridge of MCIII.
- Medial and lateral condyles of MCIII.
- Proximopalmar/plantar P1.
- Origin of short collateral ligaments.

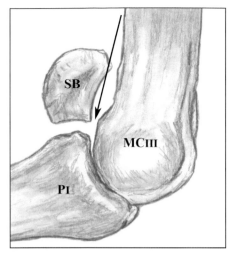

**Figure 14-21** Anatomical drawing indicating the correct position and angle of the arthroscope during examination of the palmar / plantar fetlock joint (arrow). Cannon bone (MC$_{III}$), proximal phalanx (P$_I$), sesamoid bone (SB).

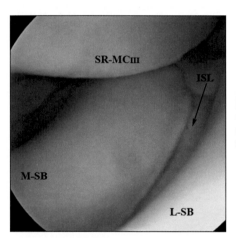

**Figure 14-22** Sagittal ridge MCIII (SR-MC$_{III}$), medial (M-SB) and lateral sesamoid bones (L-SB), inter-sesamoidean ligament (ISL).

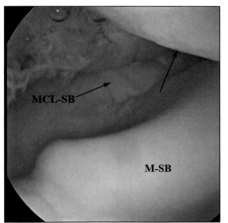

**Figure 14-23** Sagittal ridge MCIII (arrow), medial sesamoid bone (M-SB), medial collateral sesamoidean ligament (MCL-SB).

**Figure 14-24** Medial condyle cannon bone (MC-MC$_{III}$), medial sesamoid bone (M-SB), medial collateral sesamoidean ligament (MCL-SB).

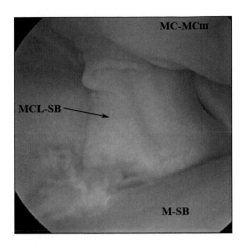

**Figure 14-25** Insertion of suspensory branches (medial (M-SL-Br) and lateral (arrow)) on apical aspect of medial (M-SB) and lateral sesamoid bones (L-SB). Colateral ligament of the sesamoid bone (CL-SB).

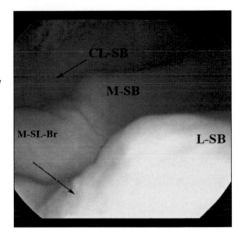

**Figure 14-26** ProximoPalmar / DistoPalmar View: Medial aspect of sagittal ridge (SR-MC$_{III}$) medial condyle of the cannon bone (MC-MC$_{III}$) and proximal palmar aspect of the first phalanx (P-Pa-P$_I$). Dorsoaxial aspect of distal medial sesamoid bone (arrow).

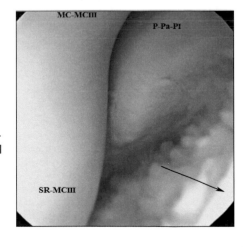

235

♥ Pathological Processes: (Figures 14-27 through 14-29)
- Iatrogenic damage.
- Palmar / Plantar axial P1 fractures.
- Sesamoid bone fractures.

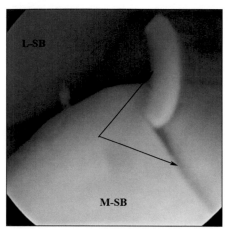

**Figure 14-27** Mediolateral view of the palmar aspect of the fetlock joint: Iatrogenic damage to the medial sesamoid bone (M-SB) after arthroscope insertion (arrows) in a cadaver specimen. (L-SB – Lateral sesamoid bone).

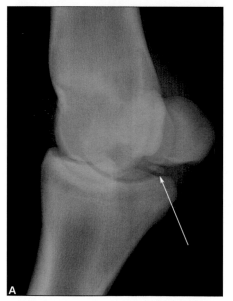

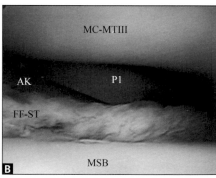

**Figure 14-28A,B** A: Dorsomedial plantarolateral radiograph of a medial plantar axial P1 fracture in a yearling racehorse. Usually considered due to trauma, this lesion may be another manifestation of osteochondrosis as it is commonly seen in weanling and yearling horses. B: An arthroscopic view of a plantar axial P1 fracture removal in a yearling horse. MSB = Medial sesamoid bone; MC-MTIII = Medial condyle of the third metatarsal bone; P1 = Proximal sesamoid bone; AK = Arthroscopic knife; FF-ST = Fracture fragment-soft tissue.

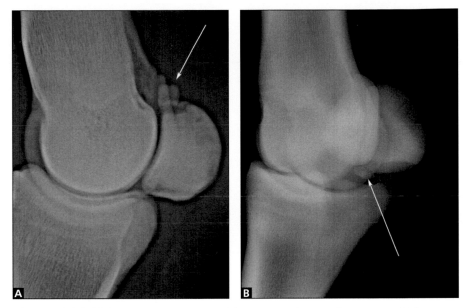

**Figure 14-29A,B**  A: Apical sesamoid fracture and B: Basilar sesamoid fractures in yearling horses.

# Carpal Joints (Radio- & Inter-Carpal (Middle Joints)

## Radio-Carpal Joint

✓ Recumbency: Dorsal.

✓ Portal Placement (Figure 14-30):

- Lateral portal
  - Between the extensor carpi radialis (ECR, avoid the tendon sheath) and common digital extensor tendons.
  - Between the articular surfaces of the distal radius and proximal row of carpal bones with the joint flexed (approx. 110-130 degrees).
- Medial portal
  - Medial to the tendon sheath of the ECR.

✓ Entrance Angle: Initially perpendicular to the skin and upon entry to the joint, move into a palmar / plantar medial direction to avoid iatrogenic damage to the articular cartilage.

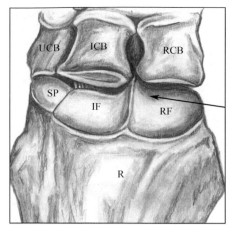

**Figure 14-30** Anatomical drawing indicating the correct position and angle of the arthroscope during examination of the radiocarpal joint (arrow). R = Radius; RF= Radial facet; IF = Intermediate facet; SP = Styloid process of the radius; RCB = Radiocarpal bone; ICB = Intermediate carpal bone; UCB = Ulnar carpal bone.

♥ Common Mistakes:

• Portal placement other than equidistant from the articular surfaces of the radius and the middle row of carpal bones.

✓ Normal Anatomy:

• Distal radius, radio-, intermediate- and ulnar-carpal bones (Figures 14-31 through 14-33).

♥ Pathological Processes:

• Distal radial, proximal radio, intermediate or ulnar carpal bone OC fragmentation (Figure 14-34).

• Synovial penetration or sepsis (Figure 14-35).

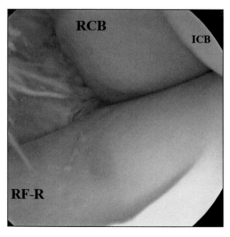

**Figure 14-31** Junction between radial (RCB) and intermediate carpal bones (ICB) and radial facet of distal radius (RF-R).

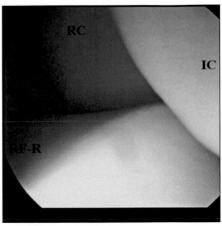

**Figure 14-32** Radiocarpal bone (RC), intermediate carpal bone (IC), radial facet of the distal radius (RF-R).

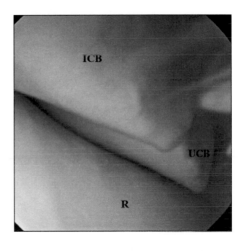

**Figure 14-33** Mediolateral view: Distal radius (R), intermediate carpal bone (ICB) and ulnar carpal bone (UCB).

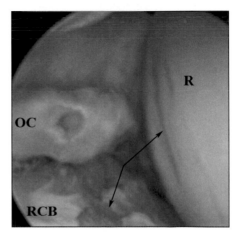

**Figure 14-34** Large loose osteochondral fragment (OC), note massive articular cartilage damage to radiocarpal bone (RCB, arrows) and distal radius (R).

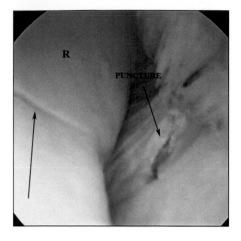

**Figure 14-35** Penetrating wound to dorsal carpus-Synovial puncture (puncture, arrow), cartilage damage to distal radius (R, arrow) from sharp object.

# Inter-Carpal Joint

✓ Recumbency: Dorsal

✓ Portal Placement (Figure 14-36):

- Lateral portal

  - Between the extensor carpi radialis (ECR, avoid the tendon sheath) and common digital extensor tendons.

  - Between the articular surfaces of the middle and distal row of carpal bones with the joint flexed (approx. 60-70 degrees).

- Medial portal

  - Medial to the tendon sheath of the ECR.

Entrance Angle: As above.

✓ Normal Anatomy:

- Radio-, intermediate and ulnar-carpal bones.

- 2nd, 3rd and 4th carpal bones.

- Lateral, medial and dorsomedial intercarpal ligaments.

- Median ridge of the 3rd carpal bone which divides the bone into intermediate and radial facets (Figures 14-37 and 14-38).

**Figure 14-36** Anatomical drawing indicating the correct position and angle of the arthroscope during examination of the intercarpal joint (arrows). RC = Radiocarpal bone.

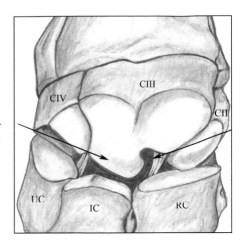

**Figure 14-37** Radiocarpal bone (RCB), junction of the second ($C_{II}$) and third ($C_{III}$) carpal bones, medial intercarpal ligament (arrow).

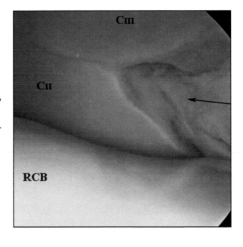

**Figure 14-38** Lateral intercarpal ligament (arrow) between the third ($C_{III}$) and fourth ($C_{IV}$) carpal bones and the intermediate (ICB) and ulnar (UCB) carpal bones.

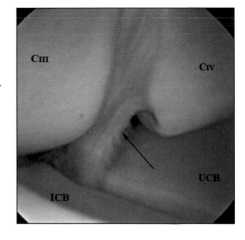

♥ Pathological Processes:

- OC fragments–Prognosis for return to racing correlates with the degree of associated articular cartilage damage. Where less than 50% of the articular surface is damage the prognosis is approximately 70%. If the damage is greater than this the prognosis is reduced to 53% (Figures 14-39 and 14-40).

- Degenerative joint disease (DJD) (Figure 14-41).

- Carpal slab fractures–Small or multi-fragmented fractures should be removed, however the preferred option is internal fixation to prevent articular defect formation (Figures 14-42 through 14-45).

- Intercarpal ligament damage (Figures 14-46 and 14-47).

- Sepsis.

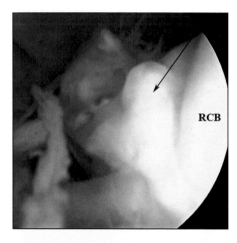

**Figure 14-39** Chronic radiocarpal osteochondral chip fracture (arrow). (RCB – radiocarpal bone).

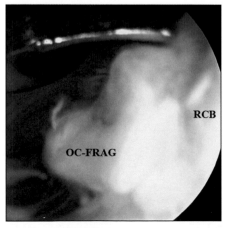

**Figure 14-40** Osteochondral fragment (OC-FRAG) removal from the radiocarpal bone (RCB).

**Figure 14-41** Wear lines (arrows) to the articular surface of the intermediate carpal bone (ICB) associated with chronic degenerative joint disease.

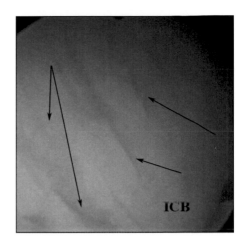

**Figure 14-42** Chronic damage to the articular surface of the third carpal bone ($C_{III}$) with a chip fracture (arrow) originating from the distal margin of the radiocarpal bone (RCB).

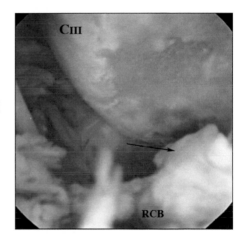

**Figure 14-43** Third carpal slab fracture (arrow). Parent portion of $C_{III}$ can be seen to the left. Dorsal is to the right.

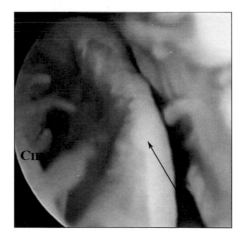

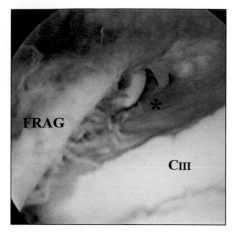

**Figure 14-44** C3 slab fracture. Fractured fragment (FRAG), fracture plane (*) and parent third carpal bone (C$_{III}$).

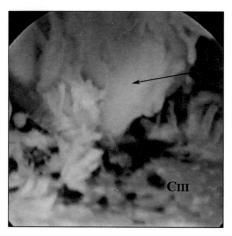

**Figure 14-45** Bleeding subchondral bone after fracture bed debridement (C$_{III}$). Fragment (arrow).

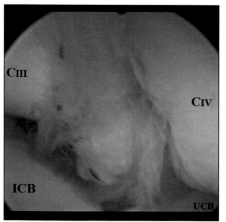

**Figure 14-46** Lateral palmar intercarpal ligament damage. Lateral intercarpal ligament between the third (C$_{III}$) and fourth (C$_{IV}$) carpal bones and the intermediate (ICB) and ulnar (UCB) carpal bones.

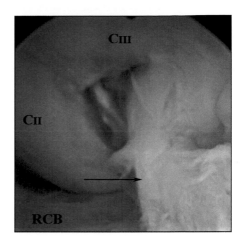

**Figure 14-47** Medial palmar intercarpal ligament damage (arrow) between the second (C$_{II}$) and third (C$_{III}$) carpal bones and radiocarpal bone (RCB).

# Elbow Joint

✓ Recumbency: Lateral

## Craniolateral Approach

✓ Portal Placement: 2 to 3 cm cranial to the lateral collateral ligament of the humeroradial joint (Figure 14-48).

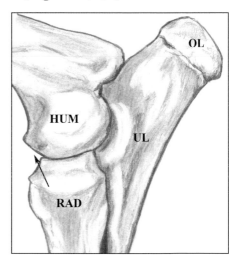

**Figure 14-48** Anatomical drawing indicating the correct position and angle of the arthroscope during examination of the elbow joint (arrow). HUM – Humerus, UL – Ulnar, OL – Olecranon, RAD – Radius.

✓ Entrance Angle: Caudal, axial and perpendicular to skin incision, across the face of the joint.

✓ Normal Anatomy:

- Medial and lateral humeral condyles.
- Proximal radius.
- Lateral collateral ligaments. (Figures 14-49 through 14-51).

245

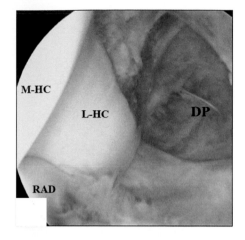

**Figure 14-49** CranioLateral View: Voluminous dorsal pouch (DP), medial humeral condyle (M-HC), lateral condyle (L-HC), proximal radius (RAD).

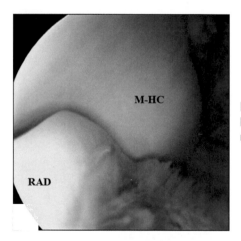

**Figure 14-50** Close view of medial humeral condyle (M-HC) and proximo-medial radius (RAD).

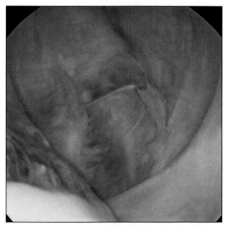

**Figure 14-51** Craniomedial Joint pouch: Medial Condyle (Bottom left).

# Caudoproximal Approach

✓ Portal Placement: 2 cm caudal to the lateral epicondyle of the humerus, approximately at the level of the olecranon (Figure 14-52A).

✓ Entrance Angle: Distally and cranially towards the humeral condyles and the anconeal process of the ulna.

✓ Normal Anatomy:

- Anconeal process of the ulnar.
- Coronoid process of the ulnar.
- Normal synovial fossa.
- Distal humeral condyles.
- Proximal radial condyles. (Figures 14-52B and 14-52C).

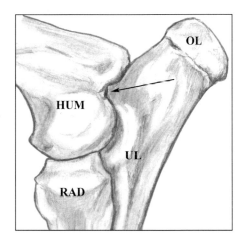

**Figure 14-52A** Anatomical drawing indicating the correct position and angle of the arthroscope during examination of the caudoproximal elbow joint (arrow). HUM – Humerus, RAD – Radius, UL – Ulnar, OL – Olecranon.

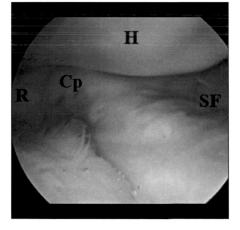

**Figure 14-52B** Caudoproximal approach looking distodorsally. Note the presence of a normal synovial fossa (SF) in the region of the lateral coronoid process (Cp) of the ulnar, the radioulnar articulation, R-radius and H-humerus.

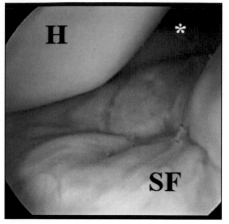

**Figure 14-52C** Caudoproximal approach looking distomedially. Note the synovial fossa (SF) in the region of the lateral coronoid process (Cp) of the ulnar, the humerus (H) and the radius medially (*).

♥ Pathological Processes:
- Osteochondral fragments.
- Osteochondrosis.
- Sepsis.
- Fragmentation of the anconeal process.

# Shoulder Joint (Scapulo-Humeral Joint)

✓ Recumbency: Lateral.

✓ Portal Placement: Axial to the infraspinatus tendon and immediately proximal to the notch in the greater trochanter (tubercle) of the humerus (Figure 14-53).

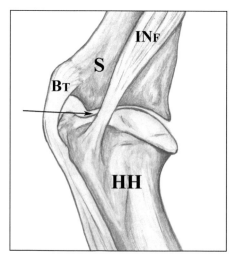

**Figure 14-53** Anatomical drawing indicating the correct position and angle of the arthroscope during examination of the shoulder joint (arrow). $B_T$ – Biceps tendon, S-Scapula, HH – Humeral head, $IN_F$ – Infraspinatus muscle.

✓ Entrance Angle: Caudomedial, following the angle made by an 18G 3 1/2" spinal needle used to establish joint distention.

♥ Common Mistakes:

• If the obturator angle is too steep, the non-articular portion of the humeral head may be impacted. Inadvertently dropping the hand towards the horse during obturator insertion will result in lateral placement of the cannula within the soft tissues.

• If the error is not noted prior to fluid ingress, significant extra-capsular fluid may be deposited.

✓ Normal Anatomy:

• Lateral and medial portions of the humeral head.

• Glenoid of the scapula.

(With instrument distraction of the articular surfaces, the surfaces of the glenoid and humerus can be visualized (Figures 14-54 through 14-57).

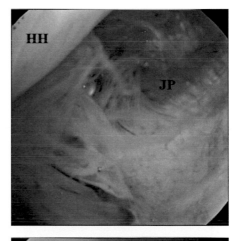

**Figure 14-54** Caudal ventrolateral joint pouch (JP). Humeral head (HH).

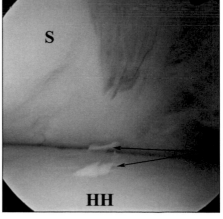

**Figure 14-55** Lateral view: Scapula (S),humeral head (HH) Note: iatrogenic damage from spinal needle insertion (arrow) in a cadaver specimen.

249

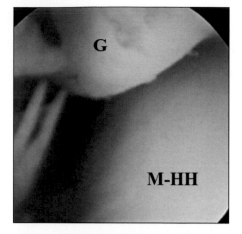

**Figure 14-56** Medial Aspect of joint: Glenoid (G), medial aspect of humeral head (M-HH).

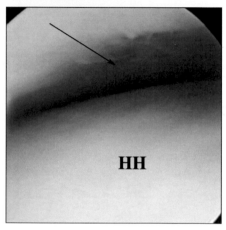

**Figure 14-57** Probe Distracted Joint: Glenoid of Scapula (arrow), humeral head (HH).

♥ Pathological Processes:

• Osteochondrosis–Prognosis without surgery in these cases is universally poor. However even with surgical debridement the reported success rate (return to function) is only approximately 50%. Sites include glenoid cavity and caudal humeral head (Figures 14-58 through 14-62).

• Sepsis.

**Figure 14-58** Radiograph of a yearling horse with OC of the caudal humeral head (arrow).

**Figure 14-59** Glenoid of scapula (G) with glenoid cyst (arrow), humeral head (HH).

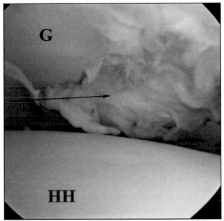

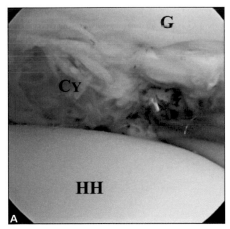

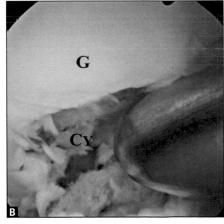

**Figure 14-60A,B** Probing of cyst cavity (C$_Y$) within glenoid (G) Debridement using an arthroscopic burr. HH-Humeral head.

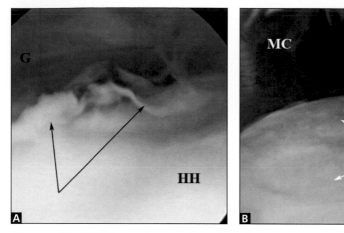

**Figure 14-61A,B** A: Abnormal cartilage (arrows) on humeral head (HH). B: Abnormal cartilage (arrow) medial humeral head (M-HH). M-G – Medial glenoid, MC – Medial compartment, HH-Humeral head.

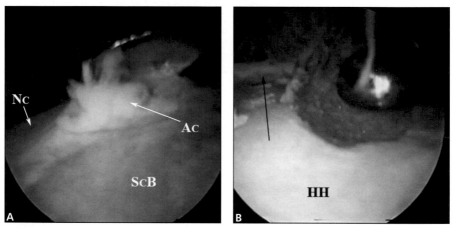

**Figure 14-62A,B** Debridement of abnormal cartilage (AC) and subchondral bone (ScB). Nc – Normal cartilage, HH – Humeral head. Delineation between normal and abnormal cartilage (arrow).

# Tibio-Tarsal Joint

✓ Recumbency: Dorsal

✓ Portal Placement: Approximately 1 cm medial to the extensor tendon sheaths, axial to the saphenous vein and distal to the palpable extent of the medial malleolus of the tibia (Figure 14-63).

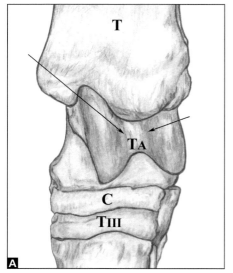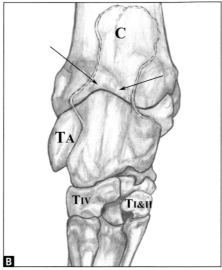

**Figure 14-63A,B** Anatomical drawing indicating the correct position and angle of the arthroscope during examination of the dorsal (A) compartment of the tibiotarsal joint (arrows). T – Tibia, T$_A$ – Talus, C – Central tarsal bone, T$_{III}$ – Third tarsal bone. Plantar (B) compartment. C – Calcaneus, T$_A$ – Talus, T$_{IV}$ – Fourth tarsal bone, T$_{I \& II}$ – Fused first and second tarsal bones.

✓ Entrance Angle: Perpendicular to the skin initially, then distally and laterally. The limb is held in extension during portal incision and as the cannula and obturator are passed into the joint, the limb is flexed to allow passage over the trochlear ridges of the talus.

♥ Common Mistakes:

• Inadvertent laceration of the dorsal vasculature resulting in bleeding sufficient to frustrate surgery. Bleeding into the joint will necessitate an increased rate of fluid entry into the joint in an attempt to visualize structures of interest. In some cases the increased rate of fluid ingress is insufficient to allow surgery and may also lead to extra capsular accumulation of fluid which will lead to progressive loss of visualization due to external pressure on the joint capsule. Another possible sequelae is that bleeding is prevented due to the pressure of the arthroscope and intraarticular pressure during surgery, only to bleed profusely when the arthroscope is removed.

✓ Normal Anatomy:

• Medial and lateral malleoli of the tibia.

• Distal intermediate ridge of the tibia.

- Medial and lateral trochlear ridges of the talus.
- Inter-trochlear groove of the talus.
- Joint communication between the tibiotarsal and proximal intertasal joints.
- Insertion of peroneus tertius and craniotibialis muscles. (Figures 14-64 through 14-71).

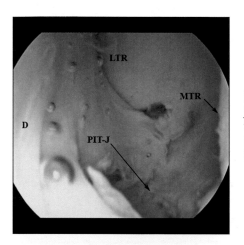

**Figure 14-64** Proximal inter-tarsal joint (PIT-J) communication with the tibiotarsal joint. LTR – Lateral trochlear ridge, MTR – Medial trochlear ridge, D – Dorsal.

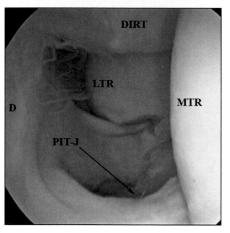

**Figure 14-65** Medial trochlear ridge of the talus (MTR), distal intermediate ridge of the tibia (DIRT), lateral trochlear ridge (LTR), proximal inter-tarsal joint (PIT-J), D – Dorsal.

**Figure 14-66** Medial malleolus of the tibia (MM-T) and medial trochlear ridge (MTR).

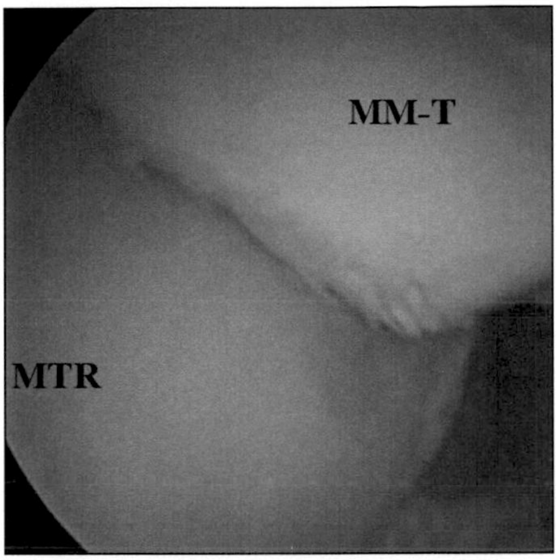

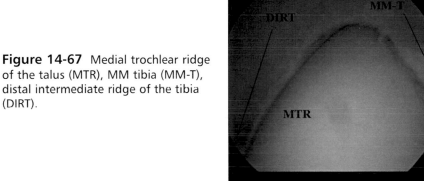

**Figure 14-67** Medial trochlear ridge of the talus (MTR), MM tibia (MM-T), distal intermediate ridge of the tibia (DIRT).

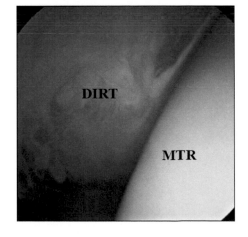

**Figure 14-68** Medial trochlear ridge of the talus (MTR), distal intermediate ridge of the tibia (DIRT).

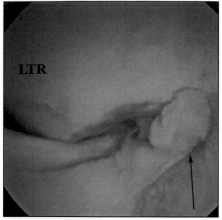

**Figure 14-69** Lateral trochlear ridge of the talus (LTR) and an osteochondrosis lesion of the distal portion (arrow).

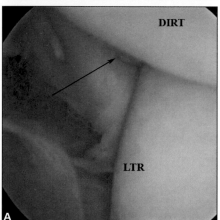

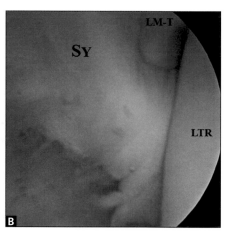

**Figure 14-70A,B** A: Lateral malleolus of the tibia (LM-T, arrow), lateral trochlear ridge of the talus (LTR) and distal intermediate ridge of the tibia (DIRT), S_Y – synovium.

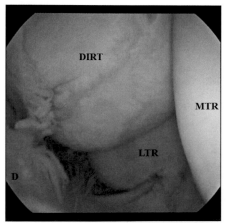

**Figure 14-71** Distal view within the tibiotarsal joint. Medial trochlear ridge of the talus (MTR), distal intermediate ridge of the tibia (DIRT), lateral trochlear ridge of the talus (LTR), D – dorsal.

♥ Pathological Processes:

- Osteochondrosis: Anatomical predilection sites within this joint, in decreasing order of frequency are the distal intermediate ridge of the tibia (DIRT) (Figures 14-72 through 14-74), the lateral trochlear ridge of the talus (LTR) (Figures 14-69, 14-75, and 14-76), the medial malleolus of the tibia (MM) (Figure 14-77), the medial trochlear ridge of the talus (MTR) (Figure 14-78) and the lateral malleolus of the tibia (LM). Effusion without lameness is the hallmark clinical sign in young horses. Resolution of effusion can be expected in 90% of Thoroughbred racehorses and 75% in non-racing breeds. If the effusion is due to LTR or MM lesions then resolution is less likely. Subsequent arthrocentesis and corticosteroid injections may be necessary, in some cases, to attain a normal contour to the joint.

- Traumatic fractures.

- Sepsis.

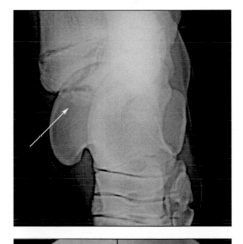

**Figure 14-72** Dorsomedial Plantarolateral Oblique radiograph of the tarsus showing a large OC fragment originating from the distal intermediate ridge of the tibia (arrow).

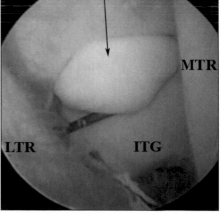

**Figure 14-73** Osteochondrosis of the distal intermediate ridge of the tibia (arrow), lateral trochlear ridge of the talus (LTR), intertrochlear groove of the talus (ITG), Medial trochlear ridge of the talus (MTR). Spinal needle pointing to the lesion (left middle).

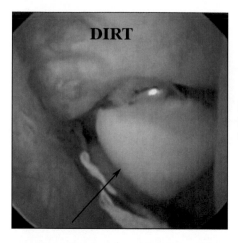

**Figure 14-74** OC Fragment (arrow) removal from the distal intermediate ridge of the talus (DIRT).

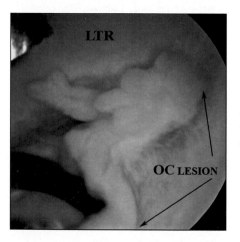

**Figure 14-75** Osteochondral (osteochondrosis) removal (OC $_{LESION}$) from the base of the lateral trochlear ridge of the talus (LTR).

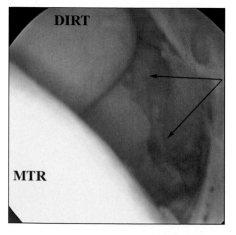

**Figure 14-76** Osteochondrosis of the lateral trochlear ridge of the talus (arrows) medial trochlear ridge of the talus (MTR) and distal intermediate ridge of the tibia (DIRT).

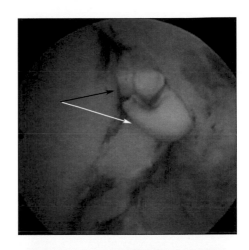

**Figure 14-77** Osteochondrosis of the medial malleolus of the tibia (arrows).

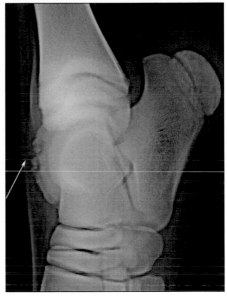

**Figure 14-78** Digital radiograph showing extensive fragmentation of the medial trochlear ridge of the talus-(arrow) A manifestation of osteochondrosis.

# Stifle Joint (Femoro-Patellar and Femoro-Tibial Joint)
✓ Recumbency: Dorsal

## Femoro-Patellar
✓ Cranial Approach

Portal Placement: Half way between the middle and lateral patella ligament midway between the tibial plateau and the distal extremity of the patella. The affected leg is in an extended position and slightly elevated. During visualization of different aspects of this joint the limb can be extended or flexed as necessary (Figure 14-79).

☞ NOTE: The operator should be mindful of the amount of time that the limb is maintained in the extended position (aseptic preparation time + surgery time) in an attempt to avoid the development of femoral nerve paresis.

✓ Entrance Angle: Perpendicular to the skin initially and then proximolaterlly at approximately 45 degrees to enter the joint and direct the arthoscope over the lateral trochlear ridge of the femer into the large lateral compartment. From here the instrument can be carefully directed proximally to travel (gently) between the patella and the trochlear groove of the femur. This position enables the patella to be as moveable as possible.

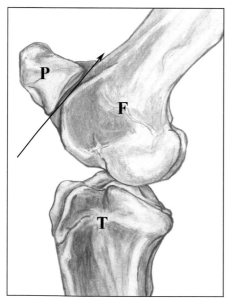

**Figure 14-79** Anatomical drawing indicating the correct position and angle of the arthroscope during examination of the femoropatellar joint (arrow). T – Tibia, F – Femur, P – Patella.

♥ Common Mistakes:

- Failing to have the joint in maximal extension. Any position, other than extension, forces the patella into the trochlear groove.

✓ Normal Anatomy:

- Medial and lateral trochlear ridges and trochlear groove of the femus.
- Supra-patellar pouch and articular surface of the patella.

It is important to remember that the femoropatellar and the medial femorotibial joint usually communicate. The lateral femorotibial joint usually does not communicate with the other joint compartments (Figures 14-80 through 14-82).

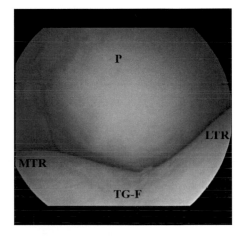

**Figure 14-80** Lateral (LTR) and Medial (MTR) trochlear ridges of the femur, trochlear groove (TG-F) and Patella (P).

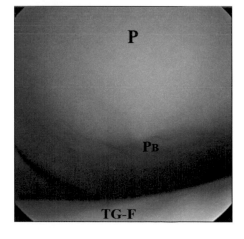

**Figure 14-81** Base of Patella (P$_B$) above the trochlear groove of the femur (TG-F).

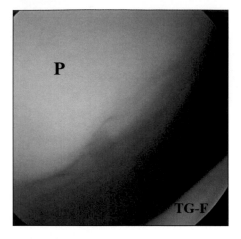

**Figure 14-82** Under patella: patella base ($P_B$) above the trochlear groove of the femur (TG-F).

♥ Pathological Processes:

• Osteochondrosis–The lateral trochlear ridge is the most common site for an osteochondrotic lesion. Prognosis for return to racing depends on age (horses <3 years old) and lesion size. Horses operated on as 3 year-olds and having lesions less than 2 cm in size had a 78% chance of returning to racing. As lesion size increases 2-4 cm and >4 cm, so the prognosis reduces; 63% and 54% respectively (Figures 14-83 and 14-84).

• Osteochondral fragments (fractures).

• Sepsis (Figures 14-85 through 14-89).

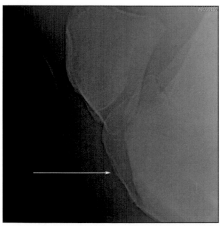

**Figure 14-83** Digital radiograph showing significant deficits and sub-chondral bone lucencies within the medial trochlear ridge of the femur (arrow). A manifestation of osteochondrosis.

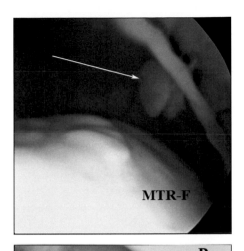

**Figure 14-84** Soft cartilage of the medial trochlear ridge of the femur (MTR-F). Note the presence of a fibrin strand (arrow).

**Figure 14-85** Supra-patellar recess (SPR) with fibrin (yellow) in a case of sepsis. Patella (P), trochlear groove femur (TG-F).

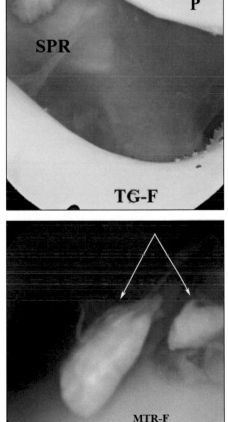

**Figure 14-86A,B** Septic Joint (A): Cloudy joint fluid & fibrin (F). Septic Joint (B): Osteochondral fragments (arrows) bound in fibrin on top of the medial trochlear ridge of the femur (MTR-F).

263

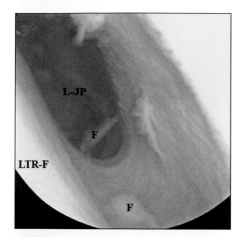

**Figure 14-87** Fibrin (F) in lateral joint pouch (L-JP) of femoro-patellar joint: Lateral trochlear ridge of the femur (LTR-F).

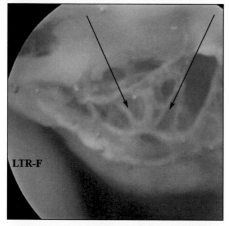

**Figure 14-88** Fibrin covering a lytic defect (arrow) on underside of patella. Lateral trochlear ridge of the femur (LTR-F).

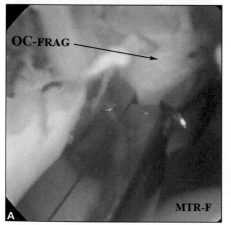

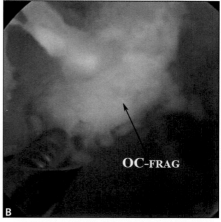

**Figure 14-89A,B** Arthroscopic view of sub-patellar debridement: Manual (Figure A, OC fragment-OC-FRAG, medial trochlear ridge of femur (MTR-F)), and with a motorized resector (B) Traumatic fracture of the patella in a yearling horse.

# Femoro-Tibial (Medial and Lateral Compartments)

## Lateral Approach

✓ Portal Placement: Immediately caudal to the lateral patellar tendon, cranial to the lateral digital extensor tendon and 3 cm proximal to the tibial plateau (Figure 14-90).

✓ Entrance Angle: Medial and caudal. The obturator and cannula will pass through the lateral femorotibial joint entering the medial femorotibial joint.

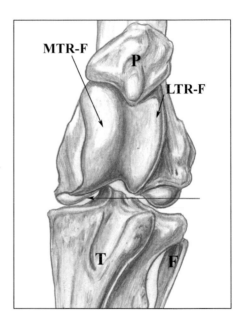

**Figure 14-90** Anatomical drawing indicating the correct position and angle of the arthroscope during examination of the femorotibial joint (arrow). P – Patella, MTR-F – medial trochlear ridge femur, LTR-F – lateral trochlear ridge femur, T – Tibia, F – Fibula.

♥ Common Mistakes:

• Placing the arthroscope portal too low will result in the obturator being driven either into the meniscus or into the side of the tibia. Either is inadequate to allow visualization within the joint.

✓ Normal Anatomy:

• Femoral condyles, menisci and cruciate ligaments (Figure 14-91).

♥ Pathological Processes:

• Osteochondrosis: Prognosis for return to racing with medial femoral condylar cysts depends on age (horses <3 years old) and lesion size (<15 mm). Horses meeting these criteria have a 70%

chance of returning to racing using conventional arthroscopic surgery. Recently reports have been published detailing the treatment of these lesions using intra-lesional corticosteroid injection, delivered under either arthoscopic or ultrasound guidance (Figure 14-92).

- Avascular necrosis (Foals) (Figures 14-93 and 14-94).

- Cruciate ligament tears: Overall, only 47% of horses with cranial cruciate ligament damage return to function. However, this is also dependent on the degree of damage.

- Meniscal disease

- Sepsis

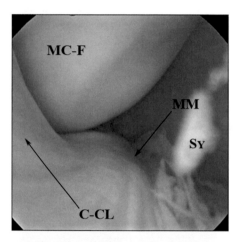

**Figure 14-91** Medial condyle of the femur (MC-F), medial meniscus (MM), insertion of the cranial cruciate ligament (C-CL) and synovial frond (S$_Y$).

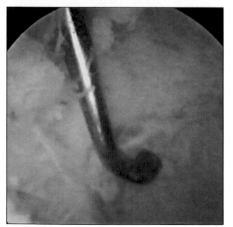

**Figure 14-92** Curette deep within a medial femoral condyle cyst.

**Figure 14-93** Cranial approach to the medial femorotibial joint. Note the complete absence of cartilage covering the medial femoral condyle (MFC). The articular cartilage (AC) has displaced medially (MED) and can be seen in a vertical plane. Eburnated proximal tibia (TIB) can also be seen. This is a case of suspected avascular necrosis of the subchondral bone plate. The prognosis in these cases is usually hopeless.

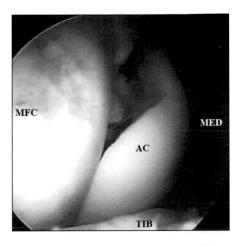

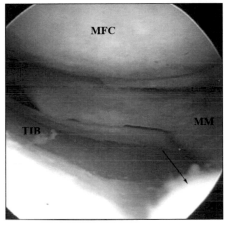

**Figure 14-94** Cranial approach to the medial femorotibial joint. Absence of articular cartilage on the medial femoral condyle (MFC) medial meniscus fibrillation (MM, arrow) and a lack of articular cartilage with eburnation of the tibial plateau (TIB).

# Dorsal Approach

✓ Portal Placement: 2 cm proximal to the tibial crest, midway between the middle and medial patellar ligaments

✓ Entrance Angle: Proximal, caudal and axial for entrance to the medial femorotibial joint. Angling the cannula unit laterally and more superficially will allow it to be passed into the lateral femorotibial joint.

267

# Hip Joint (Coxo-Femoral Joint)

✓ Recumbency: Lateral

✓ Portal Placement: 2 cm proximal to the greater trochanter (in the intertrochanteric fossa) midway between the cranial and caudal portions of the greater trochanter (Figure 14-95).

✓ Entrance Angle: Cranial and axial to the incision.

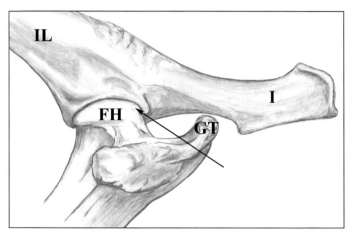

**Figure 14-95** Anatomical drawing indicating the correct position and angle of the arthroscope during examination of the hip joint (arrow). IL – Ileum, I – Ishium, FH – Femoral head, GT – greater trochanter.

✓ Normal Anatomy:
- Articular cartilage of the femoral head and acetabulum.
- Vascular labrum (lip of the acetabulum).
- Proper ligament of the femur. (Figures 14-96A-D).

♥ Pathological Processes:
- Osteochondrosis.
- Osteochondral fragmentation (chip fractures of the acetabular rim).
- Degenerative joint disease.
- Tearing of the round ligament (ligament of the femoral head).
- Sepsis.

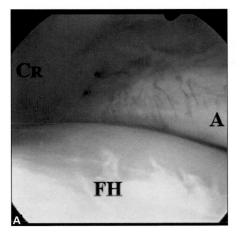

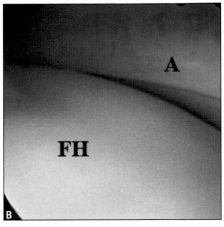

**Figure 14-96A** Arthroscopic view of the hip joint looking cranially (CR). Note the vascular nature of the acetabular rim (A) and the femoral head (FH).

**Figure 14-96B** As above, moving the arthroscope caudally (mid-hip region). A – acetabular rim and femoral head (FH).

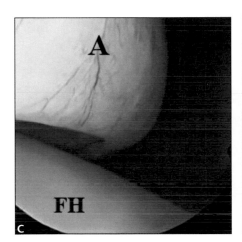

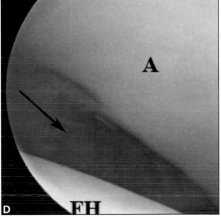

**Figure 14-96C** As above, looking caudally (CA). Acetabular rim (A) and femoral head (FH).

**Figure 14-96D** As above with hip joint distracted. Acetabular cup (A), femoral head (FH) and proper ligament of the head of the femur (arrow) within the acetabular fossa.

# Temporomandibular Joint

✓ Recumbency: Lateral

✓ Portal Placement: In the middle of the joint capsule bulge, caudodorsal to the articular condyle of the mandible (Figure 14-97).

✓ Entrance Angle: Rostromedial. It is important to advance the arthroscope more medially than rostrally as this is a narrow joint (rostro-caudally) but deep (lateromedially).

✓ Normal Anatomy:

- Articular surface of the temporal bone and articular disc (Figure 14-98).

♥ Pathological Processes:

- Chondropathy of the articular disc.
- DJD of the joint.
- Foreign bodies.
- Sepsis.

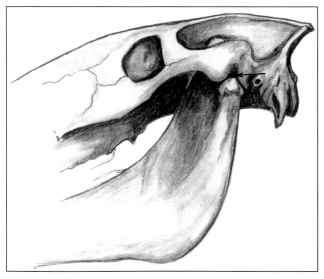

**Figure 14-97** Anatomical drawing indicating the correct position and angle of the arthroscope during examination of the temporomandibular joint (arrow). Note: Arthoscope entry is perpendicular to the skin and joint surface.

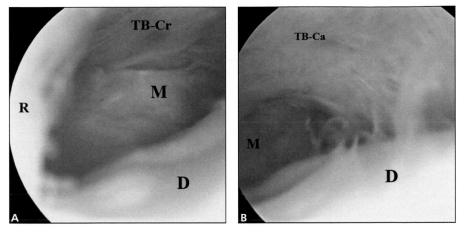

**Figure 14-98A,B** A: Rostral attachment of the joint capsule (R) with the fibro-cartilagenous disc (D), temporal bone (TB-Cr), M – medial. B: Caudal attachment of the joint capsule with the disc (D), temporal bone (TB-Ca).

# Tenoscopy and Bursoscopy

## Navicular Bursa

✓ Recumbency: Lateral

✓ Portal Placement:

a. Immediately proximal and axial to the collateral cartilages of P3 and the neurovascular bundle, and abaxial to the deep digital flexor tendon (Figure 14-99A).

b. Enter the tendon sheath (in routine fashion, Figure 14-100, or immediately distal to the distal digital annular ligament (D-DAL)). and advance to the distal reflection of this structure. Using arthroscopic scissors, cut through the bottom of the tendon sheath on the palmar / plantar aspect to open the navicular bursa. The hole should then be opened as much as possible from a lateral to medial direction to allow entry into the bursa with the arthroscope. Care: Cutting in a dorsal direction (rather then palmar / plantar will result in entry into the coffin joint.

✓ Entrance Angle: Distally and axially, dorsal to the deep digital flexor tendon aiming for the midpoint of $P_3$.

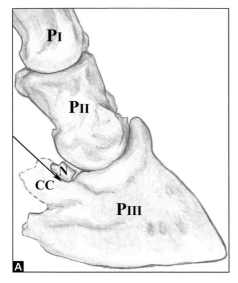

**Figure 14-99A** Anatomical drawing indicating the correct position and angle of the arthroscope during examination of the navicular bursa (arrow). PI – Proximal phalanx, PII – Second phalanx, PIII- Third phalanx (coffin bone), N – Navicular bone, CC – Colateral cartilages of the coffin bone.

♥ Common Mistakes:

• If the entrance angle is too steep the trochar will bypass the bursa and enter the soft tissue of the digital cushion. Conversely, if the angle is too shallow, the palmar / plantar pouch of the coffin joint may be entered. If the angle is too axial the tendon sheath may be inadvertently punctured.

✔ Normal Anatomy:

• Deep digital flexor tendon (DDFT).

• Navicular bone.

• Abaxial plica.

• Impar ligament. (Figures 14-99B and C)

✔ Pathological Processes:

• DDFT tears.

• Sepsis.

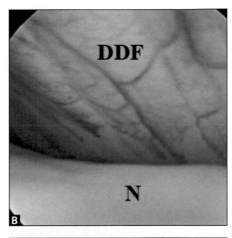

**Figure 14-99B** Intrabursal view of the deep digital flexor tendon (DDF) and navicular bone (N).

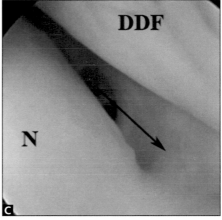

**Figure 14-99C** Intrabursal view of the abaxial plica (arrow) joining the deep digital flexor tendon (DDF) to the navicular bone (N).

# Flexor Tendon Sheath

✓ Recumbency: Lateral

✓ Portal Placement: Immediately distal to the volar annular ligament, proximal to the proximal digital annular ligament (Figure 14-100).

✓ Entrance Angle: Proximo-medially, with the camera portion of the arthroscope at the heel bulbs and the tip pointed proximally.

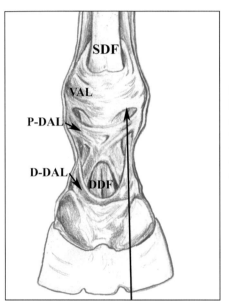

**Figure 14-100** Anatomical drawing indicating the correct position and angle of the arthroscope during examination of the flexor tendon sheath (arrow). SDF – Superficial digital flexor tendon, DDF – Deep digital flexor tendon, VAL – Volar annular ligament, P-DAL – Proximal digital annular ligament, D-DAL – Distal digital annular ligament.

♥ Common Mistakes:

• Failure to place the portal sufficiently abaxial will result in the operator attempting to enter the sheath through the palmar / plantar retinaculum. Attention must be paid to the degree of extension of the toe during this procedure, this is especially important with respect to the hind-limb. The presence of the reciprocal apparatus in this limb can frustrate toe extension and the presence of the heel-bulb can frustrate movement of the tenoscope and associated camera unit.

✓ Normal Anatomy:

• Proximal annular ligament.

• Superficial (SDF) and deep digital flexor tendons (DDFT).

• Manica flexoria.

• Impression of the sesamoid bones. (Figures 14-101 through 14-105).

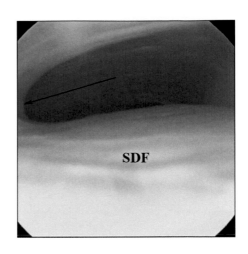

**Figure 14-101** Proximal view within the flexor tendon sheath. Superficial digital flexor tendon (SDF), normal midline plica (arrow).

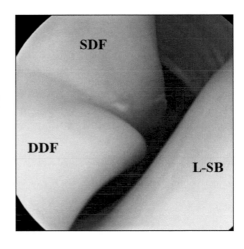

**Figure 14-102** Superficial (SDF) and deep (DDF) digital flexor tendons in the region of the lateral sesamoid bone (L-SB).

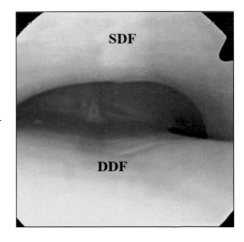

**Figure 14-103** Proximal view. The deep (DDF) digital flexor tendon underneath the superficial (SDF) tendon.

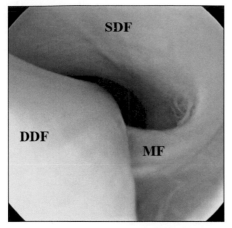

**Figure 14-104** Superficial digital (SDF) above the deep digital (DDF) flexor tendon in the region of the manica flexoria (MF).

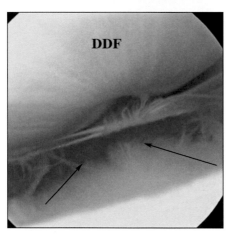

**Figure 14-105** Deep digital flexor tendon (DDF) at the region of the distal reflection of tendon sheath (arrows).

♥ Pathological Processes:
- Sepsis (Figures 14-106 through 14-108).
- Foreign Bodies.
- Adhesions.
- Tears in manica flexoria or DDFT (Figure 14-109).

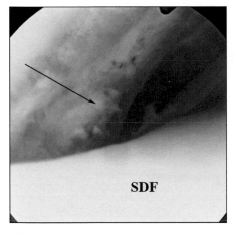

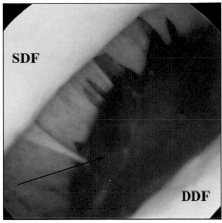

**Figure 14-106** Peri-sheath abscess: Note inflammation on inside of sheath (arrow), above the superficial digital flexor tendon (SDF).

**Figure 14-107** Proximal extent of tendon sheath: Superficial (SDF) and deep (DDF) digital flexor tendons. Blood clot (arrow).

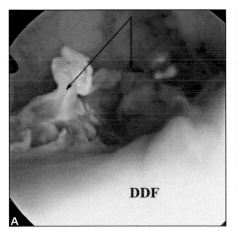

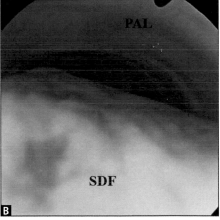

**Figure 14-108A,B** A: Fibrin and debris (arrows) at the distal extent of the sheath in a case of septic tenosynovitis. Deep digital flexor tendon (DDF). B: Extensive pannus on the surface of the superficial digital flexor tendon (SDF) in the same case of septic tenosynovitis. Note the presence of the volar (palmar) annular ligament (PAL).

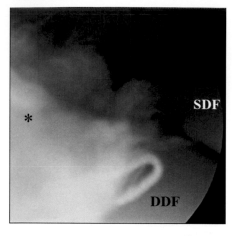

**Figure 14-109** A tear (*) to the lateral aspect of the deep digital flexor tendon (DDF). SDF – Superficial digital flexor tendon.

# Extensor Tendon Sheaths

✓ Recumbency: Dorsal or Lateral.

✓ Portal Placement: Dependent on sheath of interest. In most cases, arthroscopic exploration of these is unnecessary. Sharp debridement and drain placement are, in most cases, sufficient to effect a recovery. In cases of persistent infection, complete ablation of a forelimb extensor tendon and the associated sheath can be performed with little to no loss of function.

✓ Entrance Angle: As parallel to the skin as possible. Most are very shallow.

♥ Common mistakes:

• Very few.

✓ Normal anatomy:

• Tendon of interest, synovial lining of sheath.

♥ Pathological Processes:

• Foreign bodies.

• Adhesions.

• Tendon ruptures.

• Sepsis.

# Carpal and Tarsal Sheath

## Carpal Sheath

✓ Recumbency: Lateral or dorsal.

✓ Portal Placement: 6 to 8 cm proximal to the distal radial physeal scar after distension of the sheath.

✓ Normal Anatomy:
- Caudal aspect of the distal radius.
- Deep digital flexor tendon (DDFT)
- Superficial digital flexor tendons (SDFT – with instrument manipulation).
- Proximal (superior) check ligament.

♥ Pathological Processes:
- Osteochondroma of the distal radial physis.
- Carpal contracture (desmotomy of the proximal (superior) check ligament).
- Sepsis.

## Tarsal Sheath

✓ Recumbency: Lateral (preferred) or dorsal.

✓ Portal Placement: 2 cm proximal to the sustentaculum tali on the medial aspect of the limb at the level of the medial malleolus of the tibia or immediately proximal to the chestnut.

✓ Normal Anatomy:
- DDFT and the sustentaculum tali.

♥ Pathological Processes:
- Tenosynovitis (septic or non-septic).
- Adhesions.
- Foreign body.

# Bicipital Bursa

✓ Recumbency: Lateral.

✓ Portal Placement: Slightly proximal to the deltoid tuberosity, craniolaterally to the humerus.

✓ Entrance Angle: Proximally, axially and slightly caudal.

✓ Normal Anatomy:
- Bicipital tendon and dorsal surface of the proximal humerus (lateral and intermediate tubercles).

♥ Pathological Processes:
- Bursitis: non-septic.
- Sepsis (Figures 14-110 and 14-111).

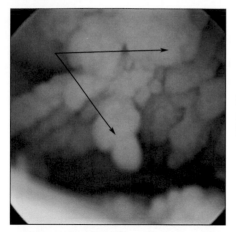

**Figure 14-110** Hyperplastic synovium (arrows) in a case of septic bicipital bursitis.

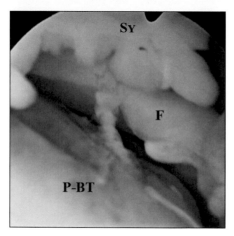

Sy

F

P-BT

**Figure 14-111** Fibrin (F) and hyperplastic synovium (S$_Y$) within the bursa and pannus on the Bicipital tendon (P-BT).

# Index

## A

Abscesses
  lung, 95
  peri-sheath, 277
  superficial digital flexor tendon, 277
  vaginal, 206
Acetylpromazine, 157
Adenocarcinoma, gastric, 143
Airway
  infections of with tracheal discharge, 93
  obstruction of, 91-92
Allergic rhinitis, 15
Allergic upper airway inflammation, 94
Anaphylaxis, tracheal discharge and, 94
Antimicrobials, 47-48
Arthroscope, rigid, 24
Arthroscopy, 220
  of common pathological conditions, 223
  instrumentation for, 220-221
  pre- and post-surgical considerations in, 222
  of specific joints, 224-271
  technique hints for, 222-223
  of tendons and bursa, 271-280
Arthrotomy, benefits of, 220
Artificial insemination pipette, 37-39
Arycpiglottic folds
  axial deviation of, 73
  entrapment of, 72
  malformation of, 78
Arytenoid cartilage, 70, 71
  deformation of, 77, 78
  swelling of, 76
Arytenoid chondritis, 76-78
Arytenoidectomy, 77, 78-79
Arytenoids, endoscopic view of, 85
Aspergillus fumigatus, 18
  in guttural pouch mycosis, 44

Aspergillus infection, nasal manifestations of, 16
Aspiration pneumonia, 61
Auditory tubes, 34-53
Avascular necrosis, 266

## B

Balloon catheterization, 45
Bicipital bursa, 279-280
Bile duct carcinoma, 143
Biopsy channel, placement of, 6
Biopsy forceps, 7-8
Biopsy stylette, 36
Bladder, 156
  diverticulum of, 162
  endoscopy of, 160-161
  opening of, 183, 184
Blood clot, in guttural pouch mycosis, 43
Bougienage, 63, 65
Bronchial disease, 98-99
Bronchioalveolar lavage, 98-99
Bronchus
  anatomy of, 84
  endoscopy of, 84-99
Bucconasal membrane, 63
Bulbourethral gland ducts, 159
Bulbourethral gland openings, 182, 183, 184
Bursitis
  of bicipital bursa, 279-280
  septic, 280
Bursoscopy, 271-273

## C

Candida albicans esophagitis, 121
Cannulas, 221
Carina, 86
Carpal bones
  chronic damage to, 243
  degenerative joint disease at, 243
Carpal joints, 237-245
Carpal sheath, 278-279

Esophageal stricture, 117
  in choke, 113
Esophagitis, 121
Esophagotomy, 118
Esophagus, 102–122
  anatomy of, 102
  areas of natural narrowing in, 106
  bloody fluid in, 119
  cysts of, 113, 115
  diseases of, 106-122
  endoscopic technique in, 103-104
  foreign bodies in, 110-111, 120
  insufflation of, 122
  medicinal bolus in, 112
  misshapen lumen of, 122
  mucosa of, 105
  normal endoscopic findings in, 105
  ruptured or perforated, 107-108
  tears of, 116
  ulceration of
    with choke, 115-116, 117
    with esophageal obstruction, 120
Estrus cycle, 196
Ethmoid forceps, 221
Ethmoid hematoma, 17
  of paranasal sinuses, 28
Ethmoid labyrinth
  endoscopic view of, 13
  fungal infection of, 18
Ethmoid sinus, 22
Ethmoidal bones, 13
Exercise-induced pulmonary hemorrhage
  (EIPH), 89-90
Extensor tendon sheaths, 278

# F

Femoral condyle cysts, 266
Femoral head, arthroscopy of, 269
Femoro-patellar joint
  arthroscopy of, 260-264
Femorotibial arthroscopy, 222

Femorotibial compartments
  dorsal approach to, 267
  lateral approach to, 265-267
Femorotibial joint, 260-264
Femur
  medial condyle of, 266
  trochlear ridges of, 261, 263
Ferris-Smith rongeurs, 221
Fetal maceration/mummification, 215
Fetal membranes, retained, 215
Fetlock joint
  dorsal approach to, 231-233
  palmar/plantar approach to, 233-236
Fiberoptic endoscope, portable, 5
Fibrin
  in bicipital bursa, 280
  covering patella, 262, 264
  in septic tenosynovitis, 277
Fibroma, of guttural pouch, 52
Flexor tendon sheath, 274-278
5-Fluorouracil, for squamous papillomas, 179
Forceps, 7-8, 9
Foreign bodies
  in esophageal obstruction, 120
  in guttural pouch, 53
  in joints, 223
  in uterus, 214
Fractures
  carpal slab, 243, 244
  chip, 223
    of carpal bones, 243
    radiocarpal, 242
  extensor process, 225, 226
  of paranasal sinuses, 29
Frontal sinus, 22
  endoscopic access to, 24
  endoscopic views of, 25-26
Fungal granulomas
  nasopharyngeal, 67
  in trachea, 88

Fungal infection
   of ethmoid labyrinth, 18
   of paranasal sinuses, 27
Fungal rhinitis, 16
Fungal sinusitis, 28

# G

*Gasterophilus intestinalis*, 142-143
*Gasterophilus nasalis* larvae, 153
Gastric emptying, impaired, in foals, 143
Gastric impaction, 112, 144
Gastric neoplasia, 143
Gastric parasites, 142-143
Gastric ulcers, 135-137
   clinical syndromes
      in foals, 139
      in yearlings and adults, 140-141
   endoscopic findings and appearance of, 137-138
   glandular, 139, 141
   nonglandular, 140–141
   scoring system for, 139
Genital examination, 157
Genitourinary system
   anatomy of, 156-157
   diseases of, 164-175
   endoscopic technique and normal findings in, 157-163
Glans penis, 178
Glenoid cyst, 251
Glossopharyngeal nerve, 34
Guide wires, 7-8
Guttural pouch, 13, 34-53
   anatomy of, 34
      lateral compartment, 35
      medial compartment, 34-35
   cysts in, 53
   diseases of, 40-53
   endoscopic technique in, 35-40

entry into
   using artificial insemination pipette, 37-39
   using biopsy stylette, 36
foreign bodies in, 53
inflammation of, 51
mycosis of
   with dorsal soft palate displacement, 59
   in tracheal blood, 91
Guttural pouch tympany, 40-41
   in dorsal collapse of nasopharynx, 63
   with lymphoid follicular hyperplasia, 57

# H

H2 receptors blockers, 180
*Habronema megastoma*, 143
Habronemiasis, 169, 185
Hemangioma, 52
Hemangiosarcoma, 52
Hematoma, vaginal, 206
Hematuria
   exercise-associated, 174
   idiopathic renal, 174
   in pyelonephritis, 172
   with urethral defects, 173
Hemospermia, 188-192
Hepatic disease, in laryngeal hemiplegia, 80
Hip joint
   arthroscopy, 268-269
   normal anatomy of, 268
*Histoplasma* infection, nasal manifestations of, 16
Humeral condyle, 246
Humeral head, 249
   abnormal cartilage of, 252
   glenoid medial aspect of, 250
   osteochondrosis of, 251
Hyovertebrotomy, 48
Hyperplastic synovium, 280
Hypersensitivity reaction, 15
Hypoglossal nerve, 34

Pastern joint
   dorsal approach to, 229
   palmar/plantar approach to, 230
Patella, base of, 261, 262
Penile relaxation, 157
Penis
   anatomy of, 180
   foreign bodies in, 180
   hypoplasia of, 180
Peri-oral axial division of aryepiglottic
   fold, inaccurate, 61
Peri-sheath abscess, 277
Periosteal elevator, 221
Persistent Mullerian duct syndrome, 180
Pharyngeal hyperplasia, 56-57
Phenylbutazone toxicity, 121
Pneumonia, tracheal discharge and, 94
Pneumovagina, 205
Prepuce, 178-180
   masses of, 178-179
Prostatic ducts, 156
Pulsion diverticulum, 115
Pyelonephritis, 172
Pyloric antrum, 132-134
Pyloric stenosis, 143
Pylorus, 132
Pyometra, 211

# R

Radiocarpal bone, 241
Radiocarpal joint, 237-239
Radiocarpal osteochondral chip fracture,
   chronic, 242
Radioulnar articulation, 247
Rectal stricture, 216
Rectum
   pathologic conditions of, 216
   tears of, 216
Reflux esophagitis, 121
Reproductive system
   of mare

endoscopic technique in, 198-204
   normal anatomic features of, 196-197
   pathologic conditions of, 205-216
   of stallion
   congenital anomalies of, 192
   endoscopy of, 178-192
   normal anatomic features of, 178-185
   pathologic conditions of, 185-192
Respiratory infection, sinusitis with, 27
Retrograde ejaculation, 192
Retropharyngeal lymph node
   rupture of, 46, 49
   swelling of, 47
Rhinitis, 15-16
Rima glottis, 70, 71
   endoscopic view of, 85
Round cell sarcoma, 52

# S

Sabulous urolithiasis, 166-167
Sagittal ridge, 234
Sarcoids, of prepuce, 180
Scapula, 249
   glenoid cyst of, 251
   glenoid of, 250
Scapulo-humeral joint, 248-252
Scrotum, 178
Sedation, for esophageal obstruction, 118
Seminal vesicle, 186
Seminal vesiculitis, 186-187
Sepsis
   of femoro-patellar joint, 262-263
   of femorotibial compartments, 266
   of joints, 223
   of shoulder joint, 250
Septic tenosynovitis, 277
Sesamoid bones, 234, 235
   apical and basilar fractures of, 237
   flexor tendons of, 275
Sesamoidean ligaments, 234, 235

gross discharge of, 89-95, 96
lining and vasculature of, 85-86
mucosa of, 85-86
neoplasia of, 88
rupture of, 88
Tracheal aspirate, 95-97
Tracheal luminal obstruction, 88
Tracheal rings, 70, 85
Tracheal wash, 95-97
Tracheitis, 88
Traction diverticulum, 114
Trauma, paranasal sinus, 29-30
Tumors, uterine and cervical, 212-213
Tympany, 40-41
  guttural pouch, 57

# U

Ulnar carpal bone, 239
Ultrasonography
  for cystitis, 170
  for esophageal obstructions, 120
Ultraviolet radiation, in squamous cell
  carcinoma, 179
Ureteral orifices, 162-163
Ureters, 156, 163
Urethra, 156
  anatomy of, 181-184
  bacterial infections, 188
  endoscopic examination of, 157-163
  habronemiasis of, 185
  mucosal appearance of, 158-159
  overdistension of, 158-159
  overinsufflated, 182
  rent or defect of, 172-173
  tears in, 190
    ulcerated, 191
  ulcers of, 190
Urethral calculus, 167-169
Urethral stricture, 173
Urethritis, 169-170, 185
Urethrolithiasis, 167-169

Urethrorectal fistula, 175
Urethroscopy, 167
  for hemospermia, 188
Urethrotomy, 173
Urinary system
  anatomy of, 156-157
Urinary tract
  diseases of, 164-175
  infections of, 169-172
  neoplasia of, 174
Urine flow, 163
Urine pool, 160-161
Urolithiasis, 164
Urovagina, 205
Uterine horns, 197
  hysteroscopic view of, 201, 202
Uterine insufflation, 198
Uterotubal ostium, cannulation of, 204-205
Uterus
  anatomy of, 197
  congenital abnormalities of, 215-216
  endoscopy of, 198
  fetal maceration or mummification in, 215
  foreign bodies in, 214
  hysteroscopic view of, 200
  involution of, 199
  lacerations of, 215
  normal enodmetrium of, 199
  partially insufflated, 200
  pathologic conditions of, 208-216
  post-partum, 203
  transluminal adhesions of, 212
  tumors of, 212-213
Uterus masculinus, 192

# V

Vagina
  anatomy of, 196
  congenital abnormalities of, 215–216
  cranial, 197